Jo's Story
Who Is Caring?

by
Jo Hoyt Freeman
and
Claude Freeman

Book Design: Patti Frazee

Excerpts from *Design Innovations for Aging and Alzheimer's: Creating Caring Environments* by Elizabeth C. Brawley (©2006 John Wiley and Sons, Inc.) are printed with permission from John Wiley & Sons, Inc.

Excerpts from *Mayo Clinic Guide to Alzheimer's Disease: The Essential Resource for Treatment, Coping and Caregiving* (©2009 Mayo Clinic) are printed with permission from the Mayo Clinic.

ISBN: 978-1480263017

Published by the Jo Hoyt Freeman Education Fund. All proceeds go to this fund. Your contribution is greatly appreciated. Direct contributions to: GREFE & SIDNEY, P.L.C. Attorneys at Law, 500 East Court Ave, Suite 200, P.O.Box 10434, Des Moines, Iowa 50306. ATTENTION Thomas W. Carpenter or Robert C. Thomson. Make checks payable to the "Jo Hoyt Freeman Education Fund."

Table of Contents

Preface

This book in being published in the form it was written by Jo Hoyt Freeman and Claude H. Freeman.

Jo, an English, Latin, and French teacher described best her reason and purpose for writing *Jo's Story*: "If you have a memory loss...maybe you can listen to my story, and it would make a difference! It isn't a fairy tale nor is it a dream, it's a story about a girl who had a very strange experience...I want to be one of those good citizens who want to improve your and my lives by helping. One step at a time...reasons to help people... maybe by understanding my feelings and how I feel will make a difference..."

Jo's Story is written by us, Claude and Jo, in basically, a chronological order of our experiences commencing in the Spring of 2001 during our stay in Arizona. On that trip Jo came into the kitchen one morning where I was eating breakfast and reading the morning paper, and spontaneously informed me she had a problem. I did not know what problem Jo was referring to nor did I inquire. I just got up from the table, gave her a real hug, and told her, "don't worry, I am in for the duration, we will handle the problem together."

Soon thereafter we returned to Des Moines for the summer, thinking then that we would return to Arizona in January of 2002. Beginning in June of 2001 you will read about experiences Jo had which indicated more clearly the problem Jo perceived.

Late Summer-early Fall 2001 Jo had an experience that she described in notes she wrote : "If you have a memory loss... maybe you can listen to my story, and it would make a difference! The first I noticed anything I was playing golf, the game I loved. It's September, the weather was beautiful, not a cloud in the sky. After hitting my drive on the 16th hole, my universe and I were upside down! But before I could utter a word IT WAS OVER....everything was back in place and I was hitting the ball and realized I was on the tee. What now?....I decided to remain silent, let someone else talk and be shocked, but none did. We finished the round, went into the club house, said our good-byes, and returned accolades with a handshake, and a playful slap on the back. No one had seen what I had seen! I chose to remain silent for awhile longer because I had an appointment with my doctor the next day."

From that date in 2001 when Jo was diagnosed as having a benign memory loss, Jo and I made a great, tacit, effort to adapt to changes noted then, changes thereafter, and experiences incurred.

Jo and I sold our home in 2003, and on August 28, 2003, we moved into a lovely apartment building on a familiar campus in Des Moines where a number of personal friends were then residents.

Jo's personal physician and the neurologist determined in the spring of 2004 that Jo should be examined by a clinical neuropsychologist. On April 26, 2004, at the conclusion of that procedure, Alzheimer's disease was the diagnosis.

Subsequent to that diagnosis, and after Jo reflected upon

tests given, and learning more about Alzheimer's disease, no known cures, and the prevalence of the disease, Jo, a former teacher, talked about writing a story to inform others about Alzheimer's disease. It was academic to Jo. Medical persons confirmed for Jo there were changes in her being. After much thought Jo felt driven to quietly, in her instinctive manner, share her experiences in writing with people who were then having similar experiences, and share her experiences with those who in the future would have similar experiences. Jo would sit down and endeavor to write her thoughts and experiences on note pads. This process was challenging for her, but she laboriously continued to write her thoughts, though many were repetitive. Some of Jo's notes and oral thoughts were tape recorded and typed with the aid of several young ladies. Jo truly believed her story could help others who had a memory loss.

Jo felt others who had a memory loss and their families needed to know they were not alone. Having perceived that, Jo sat down time and again endeavoring to write her story to inform others who had memory loss of her experiences of which Jo wanted to share and relate to others that they were not alone, thinking she could make a difference in the life of others perplexed by unusual, strange, startling experiences, some of which cause great consternation.

It was Jo's intention her story be informative!

In September of 2005 Jo became a resident in the Assisted Living Program/Dementia (ALP/D) facility on campus where Jo continued to write her story, though Jo could not write as she endeavored previously, friends visiting her used a hand-held microcassette recorder to record their discussions, which were later typed.

Subsequent to Jo moving into the ALP/D facility we continued our walks in the hallways on campus before bedtime. About the first of March 2006 as we were walking, Jo suggested giving her head to research, stating they couldn't find a cure for Alzheimer's and maybe it would help in their research. Jo then requested I determine how one might do as she suggested. Subsequently, on or about March 6, 2006, I directed communications to two separate doctor acquaintances, related to them the above, in substance, and inquired of them as Jo suggested. You will read the efforts and inquiries I made, and responses I received herein.

Jo made the transition from home to residency in the ALP/D facility quite well, especially after Jo came to know and developed a friendship with a nurse who assumed, at times, the position of an activity director. Jo and that person developed a personal relationship which greatly elated Jo. I was extremely pleased to observe that, when the two were responding one to the other, Jo had a natural elation, smile, laughter, spontaneous actions, and more importantly, Jo then had a friend in her new environment with whom she could communicate and look forward to seeing and being with each day. That relationship ended May 9, 2006, when that friend was given a going-away event in the ALP/D facility. She had given notice of leaving to further her education.

In the spring of 2006 a new Assisted Living Director(ALD) was hired, and a person identified as Supervisor of ALP/D staff (SAS) became known; an Assisted Living-ALP/D RN(RN) assumed some assigned duties in the ALP/D facility.

On June 30, 2006, the RN informed me that either she or the ALD had called Jo's personal physician's office, and talked to the doctor or someone in that office about a behavior change in Jo, requesting or inquiring if the doctor would prescribe medication for the perceived behavior change. It was then reported to me that Jo's doctor would not prescribe medication. The RN then related that Jo's doctor said Jo should be seen by a neurologist. I was not advised of the perceived behavior change, nor was informed, prior to June 30, 2006, of the staff's decision to call Jo's doctor. I immediately became aware of the drastic change in Jo's environment, which explained why Jo acted at the time so insecure, tense, and fearful.

June 30, 2006 was just the beginning of very devastating periods of time continuing for the remainder of the year, about which I encourage you to read, and which Jo would have told you about, but those times resulted in no further writing or dictation by Jo; she was then a changed person.

Experiences Jo and I had, plus research I did, caused me to write my "Alzheimer's Paper" signed 1-12-07, wherein you will learn, among other things, about Alzheimer's disease, and prescribed procedures to be followed if a staff person believes a resident in a dementia care facility has a behavior change.

Jo's Alzheimer's disease had progressed further, and there were threats that Jo might be removed from the ALP/D facility to a nursing unit that was not a certified Chronic Confusion Dementia Illness (CCDI) unit. On January 18, 2007, as Jo received care at Methodist Hospital, I contacted staff at a CCDI facility, which had opened in October 2006. The staff was very accommodating.

On January 22, 2007, when Jo was released from the hospital, she was taken to and became a new resident at that

CCDI facility where she remained until her death at 7:02 p.m. on October 30, 2010.

The day following Jo's death an autopsy was performed. Cause of Death: Complications of progressive dementia due to Diffuse Lewy body disease, Alzheimer's Disease, and cerebrovascular disease. Other Significant Conditions: None. Manner of Death: Natural.

Our experiences caused me to write a paper I entitled "Questions for Physicians," signed by me 3-10-07. I wish that someone had placed a similar "Questions" paper in the hands of Jo and myself back in 2001, shortly after Jo had hit her ball off the 16th tee. It would have been a great help! It could be a great help to you, if you are as green, naive, and uninformed as Jo and I initially were about dementia.

I was made aware in 2006 persons caring for Alzheimer's/dementia diseased persons need special skills to care properly for those diseased individuals.

Later, subsequent to its publication, I was given a copy of "The Hub," the Iowa CareGivers Association Newsletter, Special Edition June 2008: Dementia Care, wherein it was reported, "You [Direct Care Workers] told us that you need and want more education and training on how to provide care and support to those with dementia and their families."

The Jo Hoyt Freeman Education Fund was established in honor of my wife, Jo Hoyt Freeman. ARTICLES OF INCORPORATION OF JO HOYT FREEMAN EDUCATION FUND were filed in the Office of the Secretary of State of Iowa January 30, 2009. My intended endeavor, January 30, 2009, and now the personal endeavor of the Directors of the Jo Hoyt Freeman Education Fund, is to work with the Iowa Alzheimer's Associations,

Iowa CareGivers Association, and various educational institutions to create an approved learning curriculum, to be taught in scholastic learning environments, and in Alzheimer's/dementia care facilities where Direct Care Workers (DCWs) will receive advanced knowledge about Alzheimer's/dementia diseases, and be taught better, more effective communication skills, and individualized care methods. Their Alzheimer's/dementia diseased residents will then be more receptive of, and more favorably responsive to the newly acquired methods of communication and individualized care.

Jo's Story is a primer, an elementary textbook, about a lovely, enthusiastic, bright, stimulating person who became aware of a change in her being, originally diagnosed as a benign memory loss, later Alzheimer's Disease. This story discloses a chronology of experiences, hospitalizations, falls, fractured distal end of the radius left arm, swallowing experiences, declining, then limited ambulatory capability, excessive weight gain, water retention, etc. This primer, a real elementary, factual textbook could be used for a number of years to educate and train persons who now, and will in the future, in their individual practice of medicine endeavor to accurately diagnose and provide care to persons whose change in being is caused by an Alzheimer's/dementia disease.

The chronological manner in which *Jo's Story* is written may not be, in a professional writer or editor's opinion, the way a book should be written, but for those individuals whose loved ones begin to have a benign memory loss, this chronology of a loved one's awareness of the experiences the loved one is having is eye opening.

The family of the person being diagnosed as having a form

of dementia, the doctor(s) treating that person, and more importantly caregivers at each stage of the progressive dementia will find *Jo's Story* an elementary text or a primer. But the knowledge gleaned from reading *Jo's Story* will enable, and cause each of those persons to be more acutely aware of progressive changes, who then becoming aware of those changes, can and will provide effective, more receptive care.

How does a caregiver find the key to unlock stored memories in the brain of an Alzheimer's/dementia diseased person, which activities once brought about in that person true pleasure? Read *Jo's Story*.

Footnote: CARING MAY BE DEFINED AS FOLLOWS: TO FEEL CONCERN ABOUT; HAVE AN INTEREST IN; HAVE A LIKING FOR; TO PROVIDE FOR; TO LOOK AFTER; TO ASSUME RESPONSIBILITY FOR.

Jo's Story

Josephine (Jo) Hoyt, along with her siblings Edward and Jeanette, children of Blanche and Ned Hoyt, grew up on the family farm located approximately seven miles west of Corning in Adams County, Iowa on old Highway 34. Jo, a very good student, graduated from Corning High School, attended Simpson College, located in Indianola, Iowa, for a period of time before transferring to the University of Nebraska, where she graduated, receiving a Bachelor of Science in Education. Later at Drake University in Des Moines, Iowa, the Graduate Division conferred upon Jo the Degree of Master of Science in Education.

I was a most fortunate guy to be introduced to Jo in Des Moines in late summer 1957, just before school commenced. Jo was a teacher at Warren Harding Junior High School in Des Moines, teaching English, Latin, and French. Jo was a very conscientious teacher, who assiduously followed her detailed lesson plans. Her Latin class students enjoyed their Latin classes very much, especially their toga parties and other special class events. Jo's French and English class students were also attentive and enjoyed their classes.

Chalk Talk, a Harding school publication, presented to Mrs. Jo Freeman a Standing-Ovation Award for her ingenious idea and for her interest in promoting reading among Harding students. The article published in *Chalk Talk* read as follows:

Jo's Story: Who Is Caring?

The most popular library in town is in Harding Junior High. It's the new paperback library, and it was conceived, decorated and stocked in less than a month.

It all began when a creative teacher, Mrs. Jo Freeman, decided to try to involve more students in reading, especially those students with reading difficulties. She found an unused supply closet, got a patch of carpeting and a shade for the light bulb, and then she and her fellow teachers asked students for paperback contributions. The students loved the idea and brought over 2000 books to stock the library. Ninth grade art students produced a "Peanuts" cartoon strip for the door, a few decorative touches were added, and the once dark supply closet became the brightest, most interesting spot in the school. What's more, the students line up both before and after school to check out an average of 40 books a day. Library management is simple with a student committee handling checkouts, returns, and opening and locking up. No money is involved, and when a book is lost, the student replaces it by bringing another. All the paperbacks are "fun" books—mysteries, westerns, adventures, biographies—and there's not a textbook in the lot! Best of all, students are reading, reading, reading.

Jo was a very motivating, stimulating teacher, a creative person in the classroom and in our home.

Jo, our two children, Hugh and Susan, and I lived at 10 Lincoln Place Drive in Des Moines from 1963 until 1979. During the 16 years we lived in that hilly neighborhood, Jo and I walked nightly, weather permitting, with our two golden Labs, Mamie Eisenhower and Lyndon Johnson. Our home was technically a two-story home, however, from our garage-floor level to the upper level there were actually three levels. From the garage you walked into the family room; the utility and laundry rooms were also on that level. From there you would walk up 10-12 steps into the living room, on which level were our bedroom, bath, kitchen, and dining rooms. From that level you would walk up 10-12 steps to Hugh and Susan's bedrooms and their bath. Those steps were walked numerous times daily during our sixteen-year residency there.

I am not presently certain of the year Jo retired from teaching school, but it was around 1970. Subsequent to her retirement Jo became very active in book club, Bible study group, church activities, bridge, bridge lessons, and golf. We then, after her retirement, had opportunities to go with Bar Association members to England, Costa Rico, Jamaica, and other places which we greatly enjoyed.

Subsequent to her retirement Jo became very active in ladies golf at Wakonda Country Club. She and her Best Ball partner, Connie Johnson, played in the ladies Best Ball Tournament annually. Jo played regularly Tuesday mornings on Ladies Day and played many other mornings with Lois Penn and Betsy Bro, until Betsy and her husband Ken moved to Arizona.

In 1979 Jo played in the Des Moines City Women's Golf Tournament, and was the 18-Hole President's Flight Champion.

Jo had three hole-in-one experiences at Wakonda. The most exciting occurred on June 17, 1986, in either an Inter-Club or a Guest Day event. The foursome ahead of Jo's group was slower than Jo's group. Jo's group had finished the 8th hole and had proceeded to the 9th tee where they waited for some time for the group ahead to putt out on the 9th hole. In the meantime, the group behind Jo's group had finished the 8th hole, and had proceeded to the 9th tee. Finally, as the group ahead walked off the 9th green to their carts. Jo hit her tee shot to the 9th green and the ball went into the hole, at which time Jo and eleven other players became quite excited, and were truly amazed by the event.

Jo had two additional hole-in-one experiences, both of which occurred on the par-3, 14th hole. Connie Johnson, Harold Johnson, and Larry Matthews witnessed one, and later Polly Moore witnessed the other hole-in-one on the 14th hole.

Continually active, when we moved to our home at 2526 Thornton, Jo used our treadmill, stair-stepper, and a stationary bicycle. Some days during the winter Jo would go 45 minutes, twice a day, on the treadmill.

Jo was a very avid reader and enjoyed her book club. Never idle, she knitted a number of sweaters when we were visiting or watching television.

Jo was a very good card player and loved playing cards, including a game of pitch. But her true love was playing bridge, a game she took very seriously—purchasing, reading, and studying procedures advocated by authors. Jo had more than 20 books on bridge playing and strategies on her bookshelf.

While Jo was never idle, she instinctively knew when and how to pace herself. She took frequent naps and, fortunately, experienced no illnesses. She was not hyper but wasted no time; she was well organized and was frequently involved in constructive, productive projects. Jo was basically a deliberate, relaxed, non-hyper, productive individual.

Jo, throughout her life, had the combination of social, mental and physical stimulation. Jo kept her mind active, her body in motion. She walked, exercised, played golf with great regularity and worked in flower gardens she planted. Jo was a wonderful cook. She, our family, and the guests Jo would invite for dinner, ate right. We were always served vegetables, lots of fruit, whole grains, tuna, salmon, berries, tomatoes, etc.

In 1990 Jo and I were invited to go with Wakonda Country Club Golf Professional Terry Beardsley and Golf Pro Jim Eyberg to play in the International Four Ball Tournament at Gleneagles-Scotland. September 23-29, 1990, we played at Old St. Andrews, Carnoustie, and Gleneagles courses. Beardsley, Jim Dematteis, Jo, and I were one foursome, the other foursome was Eyberg, Dick Thornton, Ron Rosenblatt, and Wally Geiger.

In 1991 we were invited by Trudy and Hal Higgs to join them, Roger and Nancy Espe, and Karen and Mike Rehberg on a trip to Ireland to play golf, which we did. We enjoyed the hotels in which we stayed, including the Carrygerry House, Killarney Great Southern Hotel, and the Marine Hotel in Ballybunion. We greatly enjoyed the courses we played, including Ballybunion.

From Ireland, Jo and I then joined Golf Pros Terry Beardsley and Lynn Rosendahl, and golfing teammates Jim Dematteis, Mel Winjum, Ron Rosenblatt, and Bob Kunnen to play in the International Four Ball Tournament Gleneagles-Scotland where we played September 22-28, 1991 at these golf courses: The Old Course & The New Course St. Andrews, and the Kings Course & Queens Course at Gleneagles. On this occasion Karen Beardsley, Liz Winjum, and Suzy Robinette joined their husbands, Terry, Mel, and Ron.

These were really fun trips and great experiences that we thoroughly enjoyed.

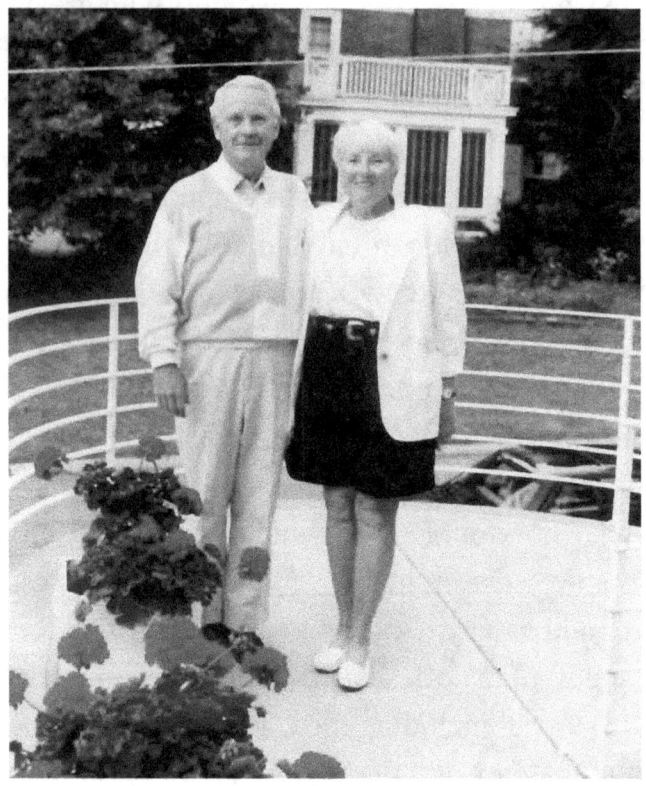

Claude and Jo Freeman, 2001

In 1994 the Trial Division of our law firm had a meeting during which each partner was inquired of concerning that partner's future with the firm, mainly or more specifically, when each partner intended to retire. I informed my partners that I would retire September 1, 1999, approximately five years from the date of our meeting, thinking Jo and I could then relax, and plan more of those interesting, exciting trips.

I retired as planned September 1, 1999. As I cleaned out my office, I moved items from my law office into a room at home that Jo had been using as an office or private work area where she used her computer. I had failed to advise Jo adequately that I would be bringing from my office a desk, chair, and other small items, which I placed in that room. This did not set too well with Jo immediately. We got through that experience without too much greater ado.

In October or November Jo and I began to discuss plans for the winter. We were, with assistance from Clark and Chris Bening, successful in renting in Rio Verde, Arizona, a home two doors from the Bening's home there, where we stayed January 2000 through March. We enjoyed that arrangement and location immensely and rented the same home for our return in 2001.

During our 2001 stay, shortly before we were scheduled to leave, Jo came into the kitchen one morning where I was eating breakfast and reading the morning paper, and spontaneously informed me she had a problem. I did not know what problem Jo was referring to that morning nor did I inquire. I just got up from the table, gave her a real hug, and told her, "Don't worry, I am in for the duration, we will handle the problem together."

Jo and I returned to Des Moines from Arizona about the middle of April 2001. Friends were calling, glad to see us back in town and suggesting we get together.

Jo's scheduled May appointments with her eye doctor, dermatologist, and mammogram kept her quite busy. Book club and bridge friends were calling Jo for scheduled events, which she attended.

Life had been uncomplicated for Jo, but signs of dementia in 2001 began to make life difficult for her. I had to be aware of things that were occurring, things that Jo could not or did not react instinctively to, as she had so remarkably done in the past.

I am not a compulsive note taker, I am a good observer, a

good listener, I accept responsibility easily, once I do then I am very attentive as to what is going on, what is being done, not done, and I try very hard to learn what should have been done under conditions and circumstances existing at the time.

After Jo informed me that morning in Arizona she had a problem, I very seriously developed an awareness of things she subsequently said and did in as casual a manner as I could so as not to convey to Jo my deep concern, quandary, perplexing situation. I commenced very discreetly to make little notes to myself, later, as new and repeated experiences occurred, I began to note them on calendars as I wanted to make certain I was cognizant of any change in Jo's condition, medication, treatment, and care I was to give; subsequently, I continued to record discreetly on calendars our continuing experiences after Jo became a resident in the ALP/D and CCDI facilities. As a husband greatly concerned about his wife who was diagnosed as having Alzheimer's disease, a disease then unfamiliar to us and unfamiliar to most of society, and not expected by us, it was my endeavor to learn as much as I could about the disease, and to be attentive to my wife's progressive changes, and attend then to her prescribed care and needs as best I could.

June 25, 2001

On June 25, 2001, Jo had her driver's license renewed (to expire July 5, 2003). The next day, June 26, Jo and our great-granddaughter, then about seven or eight years of age, did some shopping and purchased a couple of books at one of our local bookstores. Then Jo endeavored to drive the young lady to her home in Carlisle.

In route a wrong turn was made, which resulted in them

stopping at a service station south of the Fairgrounds in Des Moines where Jo called the home of her young passenger. After the call, our great-granddaughter was returned home safely and Jo returned safely to our home.

The next day a person from the service station called our home to inform us Jo had left her billfold after making a phone call at the station. Jo and I drove to the station and noticed many trucks were loading and unloading products at sites in the area.

The person at the station informed us we were very fortunate the particular young man found Jo's billfold. I obtained the name of the young man who found the billfold; I called him, then I drove to his home to personally thank him. He told me that when he looked for identification in the billfold he observed the owner lived on the same street as his close, personal friend Steve lived—a young man and his family Jo and I knew and liked very well. We were very fortunate.

August 22, 2001

Jo had cataract surgery, left eye. We sent $1,000 deposit for Rio Verde home rental for 2002. There were a few social experiences where Jo could not express herself as she usually, so spontaneously, would. And there were times when she would reflect on prior occurrences which, at the time of reflection, she felt those occurrences could have been more favorable for her—showing a bit of remorse.

We began to discuss selling our home at 2526 Thornton, and placing our name on a waiting list for an apartment at Wesley Acres in Des Moines. A number of personal friends and other persons we knew were then residents at that location. We placed our name on the waiting list after looking at apartments located there.

I drove Jo to her scheduled doctor appointment. I waited in the reception area when Jo was informed her doctor was ready to see her. Before Jo came back to the waiting area, her doctor came and motioned for me to follow him to his office. He informed me, based upon his examination, and conversation with Jo that he would refer Jo to a neurologist. Subsequent to Jo being examined by the neurologist, Jo was diagnosed as having a benign memory loss, for which medication was prescribed.

October 22, 2001

Apparently we were to have veal or lamb for dinner, but could not find it at the time for preparing it to be cooked. Looking all over we found it downstairs in the sink in its wrapper thawing, apparently where it had been placed when removed from the freezer. Later we looked all over for a large kitchen knife, which was not found for a couple of days. There was a day Jo inquired "What did someone do with my mop bucket? If I find it, I'll break the arm of the person who moved it." She reported she had lost four colored food articles sitting on the table for a couple of days. She said she misplaced the stove and refrigerator manuals; she looked everywhere and could not find them. She reported she found them on the 23rd and put them on a chair in the kitchen. When asked, she couldn't remember where she found the manuals.

We at the time were contemplating our return to Rio Verde in 2002. Near the end of 2001 Jo informed me she did not want to go back to Rio Verde in 2002; therefore, I had to cancel our reservation.

November 15, 2001

Our cleaning lady called about 2:30 p.m. to remind Jo it was her day to clean, but she found no one home earlier when she arrived to clean. The cleaning was rescheduled for the 20th.

December 28, 2001

Jo was scheduled for a CT Scan, EEG, and EKG. Later Jo's personal doctor called to report neuro-degenerative disorder; CT Scan showed no bleeding–atrophy mild–no fluid.

January 2, 2002

Jo saw her personal physician and the neurologist he had referred her to in 2001, then saw that doctor again in February 2002, at which time he reported, in substance, no Alzheimer's yet, but prescribed a medication, Aricept, to retard or delay the progression of Alzheimer's.

Jo kept attending book club and Bible study, and played bridge. We continued to be active in our investment club, Flexible Flyers, and other social activities, but obvious changes and noticeable progression of Jo's prescribed benign memory loss resulted in frequent periods of stressful tension and extreme frustration for both Jo and me.

January 20, 2002

Jo had eye surgery at 8:10 a.m. to be followed by an eye examination on the next day.

March 28, 2002

The marketing director called for Jo and I to look at an apartment at Wesley. We found it too small, and the west sun would be too hot in summer. Jo was concerned there would be nothing to do there for her.

April 30, 2002

Jo related she did not want to move and said she felt like a prisoner in her own home; to move would just change prison address. She said, "People at Wesley Acres would be coming and going, and I'd just be stuck there—same way in Arizona, just stuck there, couldn't do what others were doing." Later she informed me sugar from vegetables cooking on the stove dripped into lower pan and burned bottom pan.

June 12, 2002

A stock broker called Jo to inform her he had a stock for her that would yield 8%. She apparently informed the broker she had no money. When I came home she was very upset, contending I was unfair. She said over the years I took golf trips on her money, the last six months I would not let her spend any money or buy any clothes. She said she needed to buy two chairs for the bedroom and wanted to buy something from Silver Fox to wear to Sarah's wedding. She said I was cold and it must have been due to my childhood, it must have been my upbringing, not to be able to understand her thought process. She said I understood all other people, that I was very responsive, warm, and helpful to others, but not to her.

June 15, 2002

Jo inquired, "Do I embarrass you?"
I asked, "What do you mean, do you embarrass me?"
Jo said, "You leave me out of many things!"

I said, "Name one."

She had nothing to say, she would not say. Then she said, "When I decided you didn't love me anymore, that is when I began not to trust you."

I wrote this note later on the back of calendar month July 2002: "Now controls my time–she seems to have no more bridge on Monday a.m.–no more Tuesday or Wednesday Bridge House with Ann Broderick–recently went to Windsor's for bridge, and group was waiting for her at Perverill's."

Jo must have looked at my desk calendar, the backside of the month of July 2002, on which I wrote the aforesaid, and after Peverill's Jo wrote: "Wrong—they were at Nancy." [sic]

We had many good days. We even went to Memphis in October, then to Mississippi and back. Most people did not discern changes in Jo's body or mental conditions.

One must remember that subsequent to Jo's world turning upside down as she was teeing off on the 16th hole at Wakonda, and after being seen, tested, and examined by the neurologist, she was diagnosed as having a benign memory loss. What is a benign memory loss? Is it aging? We never assumed anything more critical than, at times, Jo was not her usual self. This condition, at times, was of greater concern than at other times.

The first medication prescribed for her benign memory loss was Aricept, the taking of which can, and will, in certain individuals, cause diarrhea.

Soon after Jo began taking Aricept, diarrhea became a serious factor. We would be out for a walk around Gray's Lake and Jo would disclose an urgent need to go to the bathroom. Once or twice we made it to the toilet facility, but several other times we did not. On these occasions, Jo would wait, soiled, in the restroom area until I could walk back to the car and then drive to pick up Jo and take her home where she could clean up from the experience.

We communicated with the neurologist who diagnosed Jo but he did not take her off of Aricept. Her neurologist suggested Metamucil, then Metamucil wafers, neither of which stopped the loose stools. Her loose stools continued and we then communicated with Jo's personal physician, who did discontinue Aricept for the time being. When Aricept was discontinued and other medication was prescribed, the problem was corrected.

January 1, 2003

Sarah, our granddaughter in Tennessee, telephoned Jo to confirm dates and times of our grandson Scott's wedding, rehearsal dinner, and other events scheduled for February 7 and 8, and to inform us of our daughter Susan and Sarah's arrival time in Des Moines to attend those events.

Susan and Sarah stayed with us in our home for those events. Jo and I attended the rehearsal dinner on Friday night the 7th. We attended the wedding at the church on the 8th, after which we attended the dinner and dance at the Younker Tea Room.

Jo wore a lovely floor-length dress, and after dinner we danced for awhile, then left for home as we tired a bit. Hugh, our son—father of Scott—his family, the bride's parents and family, and many relatives and friends were in attendance. Jo was basically her normal self during all events.

Jo and I had not told anyone of her experience or of the doctor's diagnosis of "benign memory loss."

January 17, 2003

Jo was seen at the University of Iowa Hospitals and Clinics in the Department of Ophthalmology and Visual Sciences Neuro-Ophthalmology Clinic, and Orthoptic Clinic. In summary it was written in their reports: "Her symptoms are most likely a higher cortical problem rather than frank binocular diplopia [double vision—the perception of two images of a single object], which would certainly be consistent with her noted memory loss over the past year. Because of the memory loss, neuro-behavior testing was suggested. Based on the lack of other findings on exam, I do not feel there is a need for any further intervention or follow up with us at this time."

March 10, 2003

We were up beginning to make the bed and Jo inquired of me where I had slept and then asked if this was my bed. She then inquired how to get upstairs from where she was standing and suggested there used to be a door here. There was no upstairs from the bedroom. Jo went into the bathroom and put her partial denture into a glass of water, then yelled to me that she swallowed the denture-cleaning tablet. I quickly checked the tablets and found only one empty packet and noticed there was an active tablet in the glass with the denture, being quite certain Jo had not swallowed a tablet.

March 23, 2003

Jo informed me neighbors were in our backyard, then told me neighbors were getting water out of the creek. We walked down our tree line and I assured Jo there was no activity. A couple days later she reported neighbors, five of them, hit balls up near our deck, then reported at a later date that tennis players were hitting golf balls with their rackets up against our house. She said she went out and picked up a few balls, then she asked why they would hit golf balls toward our house. Later that same day she reiterated the same story.

March 25, 2003

We were notified our offer on the seventh-floor apartment at Wesley Acres was accepted. That same day Jo reported neighbors were playing tennis.

March 27, 2003

Jo reported neighbors, five of them, hit balls up near our deck, a white ball. Later Jo was in the kitchen and said she was going upstairs to the bedroom (the kitchen and our bedroom were on the same floor). She contended someone opened our garage door, which didn't occur. Not too good today, bad recall, strange sayings and contentions.

March 29, 2003

Jo saw deer leaving our woods to go out to feed and asked me if I had heard people in the yard. She said a deer was caught in the neighbor's fence (not so); then inquired about little holes in the woods behind our house. "Could deer be digging for water?" she asked. She took a nap, then couldn't find her glasses. Later we found her glasses on a chair in her closet, clothes on the chair covered the glasses.

March 30, 2003

Jo asserted somebody was moving her clothes to make her think she was crazy. She wished she had seen my closet first (which was just opposite of her closet door); she would have chosen it. This conversation was taking place on our way to Sunday early church service.

April 11, 2003

Commencing four days of constipation, the doctor told Jo to go to the store and purchase Milk of Magnesia. I sold Jo's car to the dealer from which we purchased it. Word was I should have given it to our son. I then gave him the money I received from the sale. He went to look at the car, but it then had been sold.

April 15, 2003

Jo says tennis players were hitting golf balls with their rackets up against our house; she went out and picked up a few. She wonders why they would they hit golf balls toward our house. Later in the day she reiterated the same story again.

May 15, 2003

Jo went to office of the neurologist.

We were advised an apartment we purchased located on the seventh floor at Wesley Grand was now available to us. Jo loved the setting and the views from the many windows across our north and east exposures.

May 21, 2003

Jo went to the office of her personal physician–then at 3:00 p.m. we were at Wesley Acres. On May 22nd we did a walk-through, and gave a check, then signed a contract.

May 27, 2003

Jo had an MRI exam and blood tests too. We listed our house on Thornton for sale on May 31.

May 31, 2003

Jo expressed an interest in going to the Club to hit a few balls, and to play a few holes. First we hit balls, then ate lunch, then I caddied for Jo for eight holes, after which she said she was tired and wanted to go home.

June 4, 2003

A Wednesday night. Our investment club, Flexible Flyers, continues to have its monthly meeting at Wakonda Club. The Sticklers are hosts for this night's meeting.

Subsequent to our apartment at Wesley being vacated we obtained a copy of the existing floor plan, which we presented to our architect friend Brian Shiffler. He redesigned the premises to conform with our ideas and intended use of the premises. We mailed a copy of the redesign to our daughter Susan, who is a professional designer and interior decorator. We commenced scheduling persons and equipment for things to be done at 2526 Thornton and for our transition from that address to the seventh floor of Wesley Grand.

June 6, 2003

Our house was sold on this date; the offer to buy was signed June 18. Jo and Connie Johnson met at 10:00 a.m. for golf and lunch.

June 23, 2003

Construction was commenced this day at Wesley Grand to conform to the plan referenced above.

June 25, 2003

Jo and Connie Johnson golf again today at 10:00 a.m.

June 30, 2003

Monday. Jo decided to go for a walk then became lost south of our neighborhood; apparently a man observed her walking back and forth near his home and suggested to Jo that he recognized her and knew who she was. He said he was going to be driving by our home, and would be glad to give her a lift, which Jo accepted. After she returned home Jo told me about the nice man who observed her being lost.

July 1, 2003

For several days Jo's memory loss and attention span were not very good. The thought of moving, packing to move, getting rid of excess items such as clothing may have caused frustration about clothing, what to pack, what to dispose of, etc.

July 3, 2003

This was Susan's birthday. Congratulations by telephone.

July 5, 2003

Jo was happy on this day, her birthday. Hugh, our son, was here for dinner.

July 6, 2003

Very bad day. Jo endeavored to clean the garage; her shoes were not a match, she endeavored to find other shoes, bad experiences.

July 9, 10, 11, 2003

Bad days. On the 11th, around 5:00 p.m., Jo walked to Wakonda.

July 19, 2003

Jo and I had dinner at Wakonda with Harold and Connie Johnson.

July 21, 2003

Jo had an appointment with the neurologist at 7:30 a.m. this morning.

July 23, 2003

Jo and I were invited to Wesley Grand for a reception commencing at 2:00 p.m.

We were introduced along with two other couples who were also new residents. Those in attendance were residents of Wesley Grand. The proceeding is a perpetual affair, held every two months.

August 6, 2003

This being a Wednesday night, our investment club, Flexible Fliers, met at Wakonda Club. Jo and I were hosts.

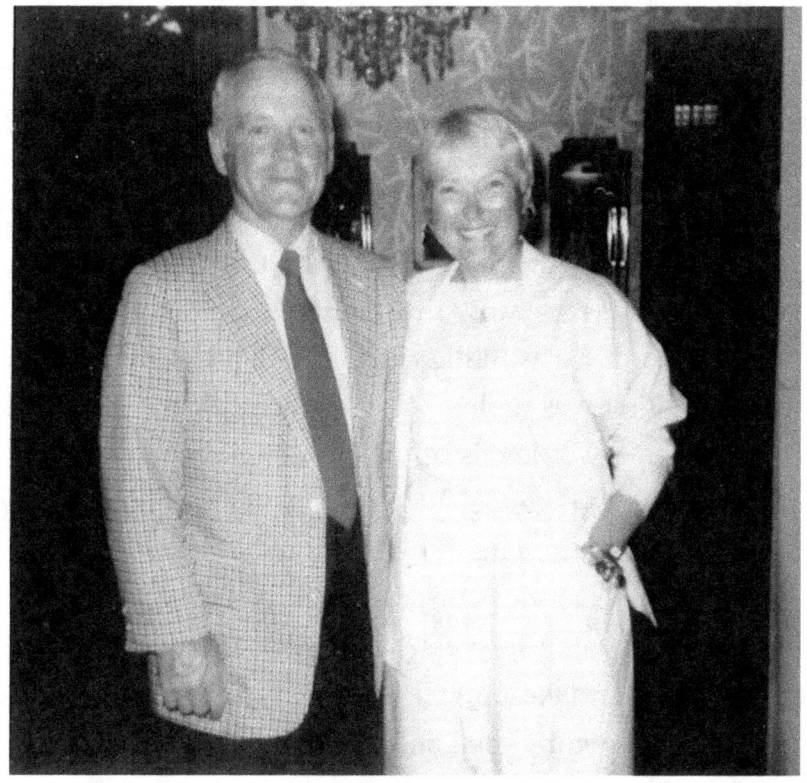

Claude and Jo Freeman

August 11, 2003

We ordered from "Two Men and A Truck" the number of boxes estimated to be needed for our move from 2526 Thornton to Wesley Grand.

August 12, 2003

Bell Brothers doing work at 2526 Thornton; new cabinets were being installed in our new Wesley Grand apartment.

August 20, 2003

Our daughter Susan arrives.

21

August 23, 2003

Susan's husband John arrives and for that day things were very hectic at both addresses. We moved into our new apartment August 28, 2003.

Jo had great ideas, and taste, some call it. Daughter Susan is a professional designer and decorator. Susan and Jo did a great job selecting carpeting, tile, paint, etc.

Jo and I kept our walking ritual in this hilly neighborhood, and when weather was inclement, and during winter, we walked the hallways on lower levels of the buildings on campus. Soon after we moved in, a wonderful fitness center was built, and varied fitness classes were taught by the fitness director and staff.

I engaged the services of persons to come to our place of residence who assisted Jo greatly in her daily activities. Shopping, closet work, make-up, hair styling, lunches, and giggles were listed by one individual and others would tell about card games and listening to Jo talk about Alzheimer's and how she wanted to help others confronted with the disease.

These individuals were not nurses nor trained to work with Alzheimer's diseased persons; they were nice, kind, attentive people who made certain Jo's time spent with them would be constructive and that Jo was receptive and responsive to them in their efforts.

Personal friends of ours would take Jo out to lunch, to a movie, shopping, or to book club or bible study, and for a while they played bridge until it was less prudent to do so.

For a period of time Jo, a former teacher, talked about writing a story to inform others about Alzheimer's disease. Jo would sit down and endeavor to write her thoughts and experiences on note pads. This process was challenging for her, but she laboriously continued to write her thoughts, though many were repetitive. Some of Jo's notes, and oral thoughts were tape recorded, and typed with the aid of several young ladies. Jo truly believed her story could help others who had a memory loss.

Here is a terse opening to Jo's story:

If you have a memory loss—maybe you can listen to my story, and it would help you, which would make a difference! It isn't a fairy tale nor is it a dream, it's a true story about a girl who had a very strange experience. I have a memory loss and I have read everything I can find on the subject. The first I noticed anything I was playing golf, the game I loved. It's September, the weather was beautiful, not a cloud in the sky. After hitting my driver on the 16th hole, my universe and I were upside down! But before I could utter a word IT WAS OVER—everything was back in place and I was hitting the ball and realized I was on the tee. What now? I found myself watching my world turn upside down. But before I could say a word everything was back in place. I decided to remain silent, let someone else talk and be shocked, but none did. We finished the round, went into the club house, said our goodbyes, and returned the accolades with a handshake, and a playful slap on the back. No one had seen what I had seen! I chose to remain quiet for a while longer because I had an appointment with my doctor the next day. When I told my little tale to the doctor he called his 4 apprentices into his office, and gave them brief notes—call Doc?-Doc..., then my doctor informed me we'd start with Alszmer....first I was diagnosed as having a benign memory loss, later Alzheimer's disease...

This just with a dream. It is September, the kind of

*weather when every golfer believes he can play the game and
today he will par the course!*

*If you do have a memory loss—maybe you can listen to
my story and it would help you which would make a difference.*

*I have a memory loss. I know it is a killer and I know it is
a killer.*

*Since that day on the golf course, What? I am I feel deal-
ing with a super power. A woman who was suffering with the
disease was Alszmer. I'm hoping for a break through–the doctors are optomistic but nothing yet....This is a disease with no
cure...*

*Reasons to help people...maybe by understanding my
feelings and how I feel will make a difference!*

These notes are excerpts from a number of pages on which
Jo wrote, commencing, probably in 2003, and continuing off and
on periodically into 2006, recorded thoughts, and related experiences, but no completed, cogent story to be published.

*A woman who was suffering with the disease was Alszmer...
reasons to help people...maybe by understanding my feelings
and how I feel will make a difference....I have a story to tell..I
want to be one of those good citizens who want to improve your
and my lives by helping. One step at a time. This isn't a fairy
tale about a girl who had a very strange experience. Read on
my world was turned upside down. I found myself turned upside
down—What now?*

*If you do have a memory loss, maybe you could listen to
my story and it would help you which would then make a difference!!!*

Long time between. I'm still struggling and a win once in awhile—Claude takes good care and tries very hard to do everything right—He practices but it's not what it used to be.

I'm hoping for a break through—the doctors are optomistick but nothing yet. I'd love to see you or hear from you! Claude will respond.

What restrictions Find out how far we can go?

I want to be one of those citizens who would like to make a difference but who doesn't know how...

From about 2005 forward, these were oral communications between Jo and persons visiting Jo, tending to her needs. These people assisted Jo, as she persisted in writing the story she had to tell, which in her mind could make a difference. They recorded and typed Jo's thought processes and responses during their conversations about her experiences. There are many handwritten, repetitive notes.

Linda, a young friend of Jo's, who was assisting her and had discussed Jo's story with her, asked Jo the following, and wrote down the exchange with Jo:

Q: How do you know, Jo, that you have memory loss or Alzheimer's?

Jo: Well about six doctors in almost every facet of your life, like memory, certain skills, I can't do them with memory loss and there is no cure, you die with it and that's all they know. It's pretty scary.

Q: Do you feel scared about it?

Jo: Well it is pretty scary because it is an unknown and

anything that is an unknown is unpredictable and very materialistic and that's all I can say.

Linda: I want to know the most interesting part of Alzheimer's disease. What is the most interesting part of Alzheimer's to you? I would say what is a good thing about the illness, to try to think of something that is good or positive.

Jo: Oh that is very good, I thought you probably would say...you would probably say getting over it which is worse, but that would sick, or what ever you say when you ask the wrong questions...Oh...and so I will let Linda give you a few final words here to make a gloomy day ungloomy.

Linda: It is a very good day Jo, because you and I are together.

Jo: You are right, now I am going to ask to have this repeated.

Linda: What makes the day good is being together, feeling happy, and knowing you are safe.

Another segment of Jo's recorded notes:

One doctor here in Des Moines kept saying it was a mild or a benign memory loss in my case, and patients could live 10 years before dying; no cure had been found so far. I showed I had it sometimes. I had had symptoms—strange behavior—a caustic attitude. My mind could not cope with numbers. I could not balance my check book. I could not follow a recipe. I could not write a letter. It was impossible to follow orders, rules. etc. As you can see here! And I was always losing things—I lost everything I owned at sometime or other.

Trip with Makenzie-bought her a new book of her choice at the Book Store. Driveway—almost went through the garage—

out to Book Club at lights I slowed to a reasonal distance to turn into the 2 Books but the next time I looked we were going to be right on top of cars waiting to turn.

The incident on golf course when the world whirled and turned me upside down—followed by two weeks of open extensive tests and added up to a benign

He sold my car, which broke my heart, a beautiful cream colored Lexus. So he became my chauffeur, and I became totally reliant upon him.

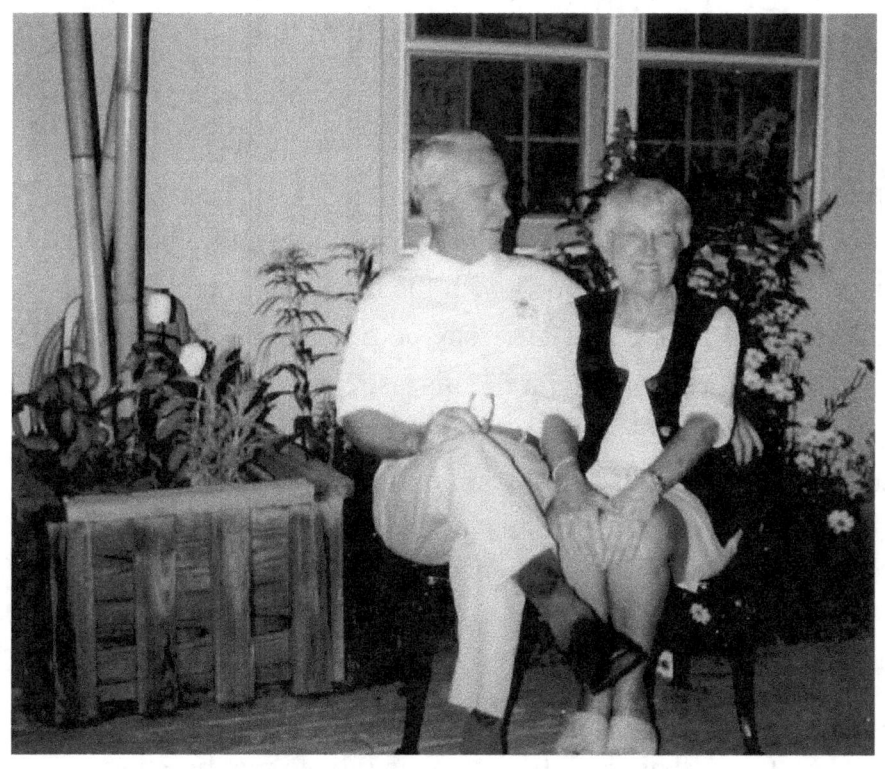

Claude and Jo Freeman, 2003

Jo answered the following questions from a home caregiver:

Q: The question is, does Jo feel frustrated with the problems like forgetting or not being able to do checkbook and so on? So you feel frustrated?

Jo: Very, and especially speech. I was so good with the speech most of the time but not all of the time. I now just stand there wanting to say this and had everybody's attention, and yet you just flopped. Oh, that just drives me crazy.

Q: You realize this when it happens?

Jo: Oh yes, all the sudden it is a bad word or you say it badly.

Q: Do you really know what you are trying to say, but you just can't?

Jo: Yes.

Q: How would you like the book we are working on to make a difference to people?

Jo: I have put this story into four pieces and...the superpower is usually developed with the thoughts of the other characters of the characters. They say no one has ever passed the 20.

Q: Twenty years with the disease?

Jo: Yes, and as far as I know, no one has gotten to 20, but I think the other day I heard something about 20 so...

Q: How many years has it been for you so far?

Jo: Oh, 10.

Q: What year did you get your diagnosis, do you remember?

Jo: Yes, in 100...well, I started counting at....100.

Q: Okay. This is 2006 now, has it been maybe 3 years?

Jo: 6 years.

Q: 6 years you think.

Jo: Oh, it is more than that, don't you think?

Q: No I don't.

Jo: I think I started it in 2 I believe.

Q: So maybe about 3 and ½ years now?

Jo: Oh, yes. That is not very long and I asked Claude what he thought about it and after a while he said he thought it should be checked to see if that would help them, but they have made a commitment and because of....well they have tried but by the time they get settled so that they could start to take an exam, it is over. It is so late, they can't. Everything has gone stale on them. So I would be glad to give my head if they could come up with a cure.

Q: You mean when you die someday.

Jo: Yes.

Q: So that people could study and try to figure it out?

Jo: Yes, see this is the way it goes, we get so far and then we...

Q: See what we do is we talk about the different topics and then we can put them all together in order after we talk about them.

Jo: Yes, I see.

Q: Another revelation...I won't let you write either...

Jo: Yes, and there is no contact between the writing and the person, you know they don't work well together.

Q: How do you get by that? If you sit for a minute, can you come up with the word, or do you just sometimes never come up with it?

Jo: Well, you usually have to go look it up because the yes is there but the rest of it is all...and I have made at least 10 replays and...but when you get through, you back and read it and you can't BELIEVE how many words you misspelled and they are little words and you have to be me I guess.

Q: So this might really be good for people to be able to read someone having the same experience. Because can you imagine reading a book where you read about someone having that same upside-down feeling. It would be comforting that other people experience this.

Jo: Oh yes, lots of...way...well I don't think I should tell you that...but along ....Susan and John moved to this little...it was a little street just snuggled up against the...where did that come from...

Q: Okay so they had moved?

Jo: Yes they had moved and they bought the plot of townhouses that had been built and so Hu, John and...

Q: Susan?

Jo: No..I don't know...Susan and John wanted to have a little relief from the move and all that and then he changed jobs that year and so they got their things together and moved there... and I had the children up there for two months... and they had been home for about...probably three months and then Susan came over here to Des Moines, so...it was sort of...we had gone out to dinner and...wipe your hand on the top of that...and then look under the light...and see if it is covered with dust..

Q: No, it looks good. Yeah, you are good.

Jo: Well that didn't over there. Then in the middle of the night I saw this bear standing on foot and I started screaming, screaming, and they had one of these secure owls...so I might think I am teasing him about it because going outside and anyway, that has been a standard story in the family and because police reported nothing, nobody had seen anything but me...but I was looking through some books the other day and beside our name was a war...no that is not right...(spelling)...w..a..I-n...

Q: Wain.

Jo: Yes, and under...we have this dictionary...that unloads certain memories of things and I ran into that I wasn't sure really what it was doing there, but for all that to be transferable.

Q: Did that remind you of the bear then?

Jo: Yes, yes...and just strange things do happen to other people.

September 1, 2003
Birthday dinner at Updegraff's this evening.

September 9, 2003
We closed and gave possession of 2526 Thornton this date.

September 13, 2003
Jo attended Book Club at Pat Baldwin's.

September 15, 2003
Jo had a mammogram at 10:00 a.m. Jo attended Book Club at 1:00 p.m. at Mianne Stuart's home.

September 29, 2003
Blinds and drapes for living room at Wesley Grand were hung.

October 5, 2003
At 12:45 Jo and Connie Johnson had lunch; Norm and

Nancy Bone were hosts for Flexible Flyers Club at Wakonda this evening.

October 10-11, 2003
Shelf was installed in Jo's shower. Jo and I went to SAS shoe store for safe, comfortable shoes.

October 13, 2003
Commencing this date, Jo and I had dinner with the Carpenters, on the 15th with the Updegraffs and on 22nd we went to the Des Moines Playhouse for an event entitled "Storytelling."

December 3, 2003
Wednesday, the Hansells were hosts for the Flexible Flyer meeting and dinner.

December 5, 2003
Jo and I had selected a vault in the columbarium at St. Paul's. On this date we paid a representative of the church the amount of the cost thereof.

December 10, 2003
Jo requested that our son Hugh take Jo to see newly born twins of grandson Scott and his wife Missy.

December 17, 2003
Jo and I met Chris and Clark Bening for dinner.

December 19, 2003
Took Jo for scheduled mammogram at 9:15 a.m.

January 7, 2004

Dick Lozier and wife Kaye hosted Flexible Flyers in their home.

February 24, 2004

Tonight I came home from Spanish Class and Jo was working on a zipper, trying to figure out how to get it zipped up. Jacket on her knee, she couldn't see or her mind couldn't perceive the zipper pull was not at the bottom. I showed her how it worked, she suggested leaving it partly zipped so she could just pull the jacket over her head. Jo fussed at me then about several things that had occurred; one recently, another several years ago, another one more recently about persons sitting next to her at a wine tasting. She then expressed her anger at me for taking Spanish. She said "Why, why, are you taking Spanish? You don't have the time." And then she inquired, "What are you ever going to do with it?" Then she contended that I caused her to have Alzheimer's disease.

As I was writing these things down, Jo came to where I was sitting and writing and wanted to know what I was doing. I told her I was working on some business. She persisted that she wanted to know, so I told her the truth as to what I was doing. Then as she looked at me, she told me my one eye was crooked and off-center again, which she had told me several times recently.

March 16, 2004

I made a note that Jo's personal physician had scheduled Jo for a colonoscopy on February 19th after which we received a good report. On this date I recorded that Jo took the antidiarrhea tablets as suggested; they are not too effective. Diarrhea persists—too many surprises, need to talk to the doctor regarding the problem and ways to combat the problems being incurred at exercise class, church, dinners, bed. Jo's personal physician reviewed the reports from the physician who did the colonoscopy and then suggested we discontinue Aricept for 30 days to determine if that is the cause. If so a new medication will be prescribed. If not, further study will be done. We were instructed, in any event, to continue Lexapro. Jo was on the phone during both the telephone calls.

March 29, 2004

I informed Jo's personal physician that shortly before March 16th I noted a decrease in Jo's awareness. I wrote the following note to the physician: "She had loose stools for quite a period of time, and the diarrhea episodes came with little or no warning. So Jo and I called your office on 3-16 to inform you those episodes seemed to be more frequent and more explosive. Your instruction was to discontinue Aricept for 30 days to determine if Aricept could be the cause of the diarrhea, then report to you or see you at the end of the 30-day period. I write this note to you today as I have an appointment in your building with my personal physician at 10:15 a.m. It is my intention to deliver this note to you or your nurse when I arrive at the office for my appointment. I note a real decline in my wife's cognitive power. There is a notable difference in her demeanor; her energy level is lower too. I did not feel it prudent to wait two more weeks to report my observations to you.

"Bathroom experiences since 3/16/04 have been: 3/17/04, no bowel movement; 3/18, had to leave band concert at 7:30

p.m. for diarrhea; 3/19, no bowel movement; 3/20, soft bowel movement, 8:00 p.m.; 3/21, early a.m., firm stool, 11:30 a.m., loose stool, 5:00 p.m., firm stool; 3/22, 7:00 a.m., firm stool, 8:15 a.m., loose stool; 3/23, no bowel movement; 3/24, no bowel movement; 3/25, 7:30 a.m., small bowel movement, 9:00 a.m., firm bowel movement, two small bowel movements late afternoon; 3/26, no bowel movement; 3/27, 7:30 a.m., bowel movement, 7:00 p.m., loose stool; 3/28, mid-a.m., regular bowel movement."

Jo's personal physician telephoned the neurologist regarding the status and regarding neuro-psych test and regarding Aricept and Namenda. Later, Jo's physician called, had a visit with the neurologist who agreed to do a psych test, which will be scheduled. We will be called regarding the date. I am to pick up a sample pack and instructions to commence Namenda. The neurologist wants to see Jo in 30 days.

April 26, 2004

Neuropsychological Examination 4-26-04 Report and Diagnoses:

Jo Freeman presents with a three-four year history of progressive memory loss and cognitive decline. Her husband first noticed difficulties in the year 2000, with symptoms of mild forgetfulness and disorganization emerging. These problems have advanced over the last two years, and she exhibits severe difficulties in orientation, recall of recent events, calculation, and planning. There is no evidence of significant personality change, erratic behavior, or prominent mood-related disturbance.

The present neuropsychological assessment revealed severe defects in complex mental tracking, visual-spatial skills, speeded visuomotor coordination, and orientation, with milder but clinically significant impairments in verbal anterograde memory. These difficulties occur in the context of a presumably much higher than average level of pre-morbid intellectual functioning. Insight concerning the nature of difficulties is poor. A psychological assessment failed to reveal evidence of significant mood-related disturbance, although mild depression is suggested by symptoms such as feelings of emptiness, boredom, and restlessness. There is no evidence of suicidal, homicidal, or paranoid ideation, and thought processes are logical and goal-directed. In sum, results and history are consistent with a primary demential syndrome such as Alzheimer's disease in the relatively early stages, with small vessel ischemic change contributing to the clinical picture to a mild extent. Her particular pattern raises suspicion there has been a mild attenuation of cognitive decline with the treatment of Aricept and memantine. This point notwithstanding, further neuropsychological decline is expected and will necessitate greater degrees of assistance and supervision in the future.

Relevant diagnoses include:

Axis I: Dementia referable to a condition specified elsewhere (moderate)…Depressive Disorder (mild)

Axis II: none

Axis III: Alzheimer's disease…Mild traumatic brain injury (remote)

Axis IV: Psychosocial and environment problems: none identified

Axis V: GAF (current)=60; moderate symptoms affecting adaptive functioning

Recommendations included:

Continue Aricept and memantine; husband questions whether Aricept is contribution to recurrent diarrhea and would like to discuss issue with a physician. Mrs. Freeman was encouraged to continue her physically and socially active lifestyle. Continue treatment with Lexapro or similar agent to combat mild depression.

The above report was directed to Jo's treating physician on April 27, 2004, and a copy to the neurologist who, at the outset, Jo was referred to, and who diagnosed Benign Memory Loss.

June 2, 2004
Wednesday, Jo and Claude Freeman host the Flexible Flyer regular monthly meeting at Wakonda Club.

June 10, 2004
Jo's personal physician scheduled an appointment with a neurologist for July 2 at 8:40 a.m.

July 31, 2004
Saturday, Jo fell, has pain in ribs lower right.

August 7, 2004
Saturday. We went to the Methodist ER, test okay. Jo was given a shot for pain, Percocet, and Oxycodone was given to relieve severe pain.

August 9, 2004
Called because Jo had become woozy, now give pill every six hours, maybe one-half pill. Keep lungs filled, walk, keep pain at a minimum.

August 10, 2004
Bad day. Dressing experience.

August 11, 2004
Really bad day—wet panties—clothing—Jo wanted to deliver a note to her lawyer who came to Wesley Grand, but she couldn't remember why she wanted to see him once he arrived.

August 12, 2004
Slept till 8:20 a.m. since she lost two days with things

going bad she thinks me or doctor should note changes and write a book.

November 4, 2004

Book Club, Mary Gordon.

November 8, 2004

Book Club, Martha Hippee.

November 9, 2004

Jo and Claude appointments with Dr. Ceilley, 1:45 p.m.

December 13, 2004

Book Club, Joan Boldt.

December 17, 2004

Jo planned a 60th birthday celebration at the Chamberlain Mansion for our son Hugh Hobson, whose birthday is on December 17. Jo and I met with the Food Director, at which meeting Jo and the Food Director discussed and agreed to the menu and services Jo requested for family, relatives, and friends of Hugh. All were here. Jo, the great planner and hostess, was dressed in a lovely, navy blue evening attire. After dinner it came time for me to give a chronology from age 12, when I first met Hugh up to current age 60. I was quite lengthy, and Jo very politely, in a soft voice, but heard by most, informed me, in substance, "your time is up, you have three minutes," at which all attending smiled and then chuckled, as I said, "Thank you Madam Chairman..."

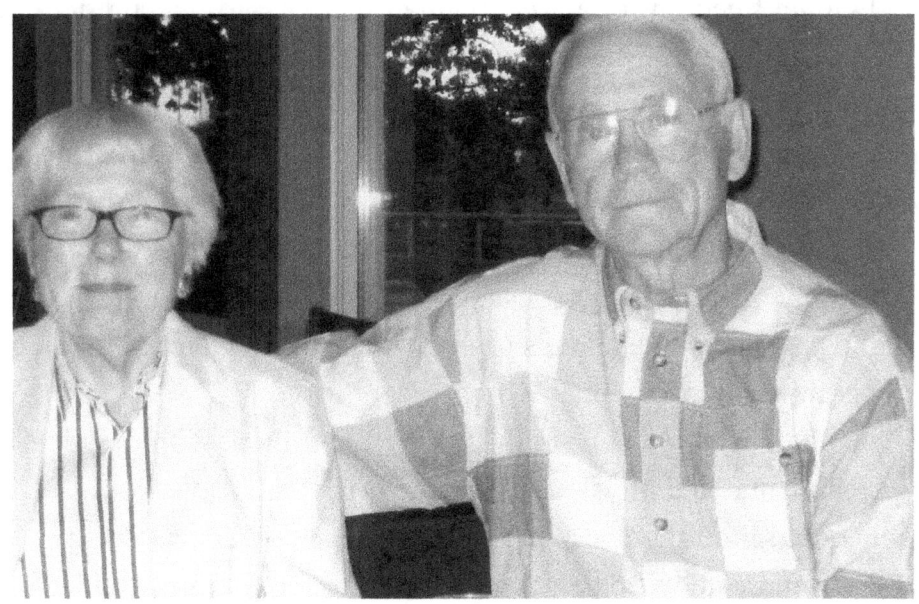

Jo and Claude Freeman

<u>The Assited Living Facility</u>

Approximately two years after we moved into our seventh-floor apartment at Wesley Acres, I had to make a very serious decision. My research—reading extensively published materials about the progression of Alzheimer's disease, caregiving in early stages and then later stages of the disease—caused me to determine it would be best for Jo and for me to place Jo in a certified ALP/D (Assisted Living Program/Dementia) facility.

Jo became a resident in the ALP/D facility in mid-September 2005. From that date Jo made the transition, from home-life premises that she shared only with me, where just the two of us controlled the environment, and where Jo enjoyed individual freedom for a great number of years, to a secured premises, in a controlled environment, in which Jo soon learned she had little or no individual, personal control or freedom.

Jo made that transition quite well, though there were times when she became bored. Jo knew none of the other eighteen residents housed in the facility prior to her arrival, nor did she know any of the staff persons there. Jo is quite personable, and in the past had made friends easily, which Jo endeavored to do in her new environment.

There were persons in that new environment with greatly varied mental and physical capacity, which conditions could and would limit their responses to a new person endeavoring to communicate with them. Jo, I would be sure, might wonder at times why I had placed here there. Jo was not, at the time, accustomed to regimentation; she now was being supervised by persons she knew nothing about; people who got her out of bed, informed her when she would be bathed, dressed, fed prepared food (which someone else chose and prepared), at a table generally selected by staff, where there might be persons Jo did not really know. I do not believe Jo had a choice as to which table or with whom she would have preferred to sit.

Some of the other eighteen residents used walkers that they would place alongside their chair or in close proximity to the table. A number of the other residents had hearing aids, some visual limitations, all of which usually resulted in a limited or non-communicative, relaxed dining experience.

After Jo became a resident of the ALP/D facility, the two of us continued our walks in the halls until shortly before January 18, 2007.

Fortunately, Jo came to know a staff person who had recreational and activity programs, or periods, at which most residents were present and participated in, and enjoyed, because of that staff person's animated, enthusiastic approach. Jo and that staff person developed a personal relationship, which greatly elated Jo. I was extremely pleased that when the two were responding one to the other, I saw and observed Jo's natural, elation, smile, laughter, spontaneous actions, and, more important, Jo then had a friend in her new environment with whom she could communicate with and look forward to seeing and being with each day.

That relationship would end soon. Jo's new friend disclosed she was going to quit her employment to return to school to pursue further education, which we were saddened to hear, but pleased she would pursue further education.

May 9, 2006

On May 9, 2006, a Tuesday, at 3:00 p.m. there was a going-away party for that activity director, an event which Jo and I attended. The departure of that activity director left a great void, which was not filled. Jo became noticeably sad; she missed her newly acquired friend. Jo did not go to exercise class–too tired. Later she expressed many things she regretted, which I knew was not good; I attempted to get her to think about good things, not dwell on the past. She continued to say she was tired. She asked me to call her brother, who then had been dead for a period of time.

Upon reflection, Jo was the spark of the ALP/D facility. In the spring of 2006 her rapport with the activity director was great, she was her natural self, highly animated, laughing and giggling and enjoying mostly the communication with the activity director, and movement activities such as tossing the very soft air-filled lightweight ball, catching the same, and, on occasion, Jo would elect to kick the ball back to the activity director. During this period of time Jo was highly motivated. Too bad that person elected to discontinue her employment at the ALP/D facility where Jo was a resident.

Jo caused me to realize the benefits of a good activity director as we struggled through several months of unnecessary stress.

Subsequent to May 9, 2006, the date of the going-away event for Jo's friend, there was a notable change in Jo's energy level, and her normal elation. I then presumed the absence of her new friend had saddened her.

May 28, 2006

On May 28 our son Hugh, Jo, and I drove to the Nodaway Cemetery with flowers for Jo's family gravesites, after which we had lunch with Jo's sister-in-law Ruth and her son Clyde; his son Jess and wife Darcy came by for a short while, after which the three of us drove by and stopped at the Hoyt farm. After that we returned to Des Moines, at which time Jo returned to the care facility.

June 4, 2006

Our friend Deb, after running the Dam-to-Dam Race on Saturday, came to see Jo to visit and talk about the paper Jo was writing about her Alzheimer's experiences, with which Deb had been assisting Jo.

June 8, 2006

On the 8th I took Jo for a scheduled eye exam. There were no changes. On the 11th Deb came to visit and assist Jo with her paper. On the 12th Jo and her long-time friend Connie Johnson went out to lunch. On the 13th Jo and I went to our dentist for scheduled appointments for tooth cleaning and checkups. The dentist said we were doing a good job on Jo's teeth.

June 22, 2006

I arrived at Jo's place of residency about 12:30 p.m. as Jo had a hair appointment at 1:15 p.m. When I arrived I saw a be-fuddled Jo in a bath robe being assisted to a table for her lunch. I elected not to go to the table, indicating to a staff person that I would sit in the lounge area. While I was sitting there a very capable, conscientious Certified Nursing Assistant (CNA) staff person came and informed me that Jo had soiled her pants, and she, the CNA, had taken Jo's pants to put them in the washer. While the CNA was there, Jo, who had no pants on, left her room with a hanger in her hand.

It was reported that Jo and another resident then had a scuf-fle in the hallway near the kitchen; it was further reported that the staff had to break it up. The other resident was a former mis-sionary; very quiet, and passive, and not very perceptive at that stage of being. When she saw Jo with no pants on and a hanger in her hands, what was the other resident's perception? Did she perceive Jo needed help in finding her room, or getting dressed, or getting clothes to put on? Did that person attempt to take Jo by the hand to assist her? Was there then a mere tug-of-war for the hanger? Why was Jo left in her room with no pants on? Did Jo leave her room to find the CNA who took her pants to wash, or looking for the other staff person then on duty? Most of the day, there were only two staff persons to nineteen residents.

It would seem most probable that Jo was looking for the CNA to help her find her pants, or in the alternative help her find a pair of pants to put on.

Jo and I went to the scheduled hair appointment. Jo never said anything about the incident, and I didn't ask Jo anything about it. I presumed the CNA wanted me to know immediately upon my arrival why Jo was late eating her lunch.

Four days later a CNA on the 3-11 p.m. shift wrote a report, in substance, that at or during the dinner process, Jo caused the table to move, which resulted in another person's glass to spill, at which time Jo laughed evil. I was not told of that incident that night by the staff. After I arrived, Jo and I attended a scheduled event. When getting Jo ready for bed that evening she was very critical of things at the facility.

June 30, 2006

For some reason Jo slept late; when I arrived Jo was sitting at the breakfast table, the Certified Medication Aide (CMA) reported Jo would not take her pills. I talked with Jo; she took one pill, but would not take the other two. The CMA inquired if I wanted her to try again, I said no. The CMA asked if I wanted to give the pills back to her, and I said no. I then went to the office of a person who had a good relationship with Jo. I informed that person of my observations, my endeavor, at which time I gave the remaining two pills to that person. She left her office, went down to Jo's residency, talked briefly with Jo, who then took the two pills.

Later, on the same day, a person, whose title I did not know at the time, but now know her title then was Assisted Living – ALP/D Registered Nurse (RN), informed me that either she or the Director of Assisted Living had called the office of Jo's personal physician, and Jo's alleged agitation and aggressiveness toward staff was reported. It was requested, or inquired, if Jo's personal physician would prescribe medication for Jo's so-called aggression. It was then reported to me that the doctor would not prescribe the medication, but that Jo should be seen by a named neurologist.

July 2, 2006

On this Sunday we went to church service and then I had lunch in the ALP/D facility with Jo after which she was very tired. She then took a nap and I went home.

About 5:30 p.m. I was called by a nurse who reported to me Jo's high blood pressure and lethargic appearance. I immediately went to Jo's facility, and found Jo very sad, glad to see me, and very affectionate. The nurse, Jo, and I talked about conditions and options and then the nurse left. Jo and I visited. I then put Jo to bed as usual. Jo talked about death.

The next day, the 3rd, was our daughter Susan's birthday, whom we called with happy wishes. Connie, Jo's friend, came to visit and Deb called Jo. That evening Jo had me call her sister Jeanette.

July 5, 2006

Jo's birthday! Susan called; Connie came over to assist as Jo tried on four pairs of pants I had purchased. I purchased a chocolate cake to be cut at conclusion of the facility noon meal. The lady then in charge of programs at the facility had placed candles on the cake, Happy Birthday was sung, then the cake was cut and served as dessert to all residents eating lunch, as well as the staff.

July 6, 2006

The RN had requested we meet.

On July 6, 2006, I met with the RN referenced above concerning a demand that Jo go to a doctor for an examination for reported agitation and the request for medication to be prescribed to control the reported agitation. I tried to explain to that person that since the activity director had resigned to return to school there had been a big void in Jo's daily activities–that she was bored, and that Jo didn't want to be treated like a third-grader by a staff person. I went on to say if Jo's personal physician felt medication was needed for agitation that physician would prescribe it and would not refer Jo to a neurologist just for that single purpose. I also suggested that if Jo's doctor thought there was a new problem, Jo's doctor would have made an appointment for Jo with a neurologist and sent her personal file over rather than sending word through staff that had called the office to inform Jo's husband to call and make the appointment. I suggested that my calling would probably result in obtaining an appointment more than a month away, and according to reports this was an immediate concern to be addressed.

I also advised the RN that a staff person had been attempting to organize programs for residents. Jo had a very good relationship with that individual, but it just happened that person had been on vacation just after assuming the responsibility as director of activities. Fortunately, after my visit with the RN, I thought that person had the same train of thought I did, namely that time would be given for the newly appointed, temporary director of activities to get things rolling to see if that person's presence filled the void Jo had after the previous activity director had left. This RN then said she would talk to the Assisted Living Director (ALD) and relate to her my thoughts. The RN met with her director about our conversation.

ALD apparently formed the opinion that I refused to call the neurologist to make an appointment for Jo. Then someone called Jo's personal physician and related to that physician something that allegedly caused her physician or someone from that office to say, "if Mr. Freeman doesn't follow my advice he can get another doctor for his wife."

July 9, 2006

Two days later Jo and I went to church services, after which we went into the courtyard of the facility to sit and look at pretty flowers and talk. Jo requested that I have lunch with her at the facility, which I did. During lunch the ALD came to the table where Jo and I were eating lunch, gave me a big "Hello, Claude," a big "Hello" to Jo, "How are you?" We talked about being in the courtyard after church. The ALD then animatedly said to Jo, "Tomorrow you and I are going to do something. Shall we go into the courtyard in the morning? We will do that."

July 10, 2006

The ALD called me fairly early and said that she and the RN would like to meet with me this date. I said I guess the afternoon would be best as "you had basically made arrangements to take my wife and the other lady you invited to the Courtyard this morning." The ALD then responded by saying something along the lines that she couldn't or might not be able to do that now. I was thinking to myself how could a person responsible for the care and treatment of Alzheimer's patients be so cavalier, and so easily avoid an agreement or an offer to take two residents out for a trip the ALD herself proposed. I then suggested I would be free at 3:00 p.m., which time was agreeable with ALD. I didn't suggest a morning hour, for obvious reasons

At 3:00 p.m. the ALD began by informing me that since I refused to call the neurologist for an appointment she had conferred with the director of the campus where the care facility is located who was alleged to have said, in substance, "Get something done to protect the staff and residents."

ALD then related that she had called Jo's personal physician's office. She informed whomever she talked to of instances where Jo had exhibited behavior about which there was concern and for which they wanted the doctor to prescribe medication. ALD then, in a near tirade, said, in substance, that if I didn't follow the doctor's suggestion to call and make an appointment for Jo with the neurologist, Jo would be discharged from the ALP/D facility.

I then requested that ALD tell me exactly what she had told the director of the campus facility and what she had told the person at Jo's personal physician's office. She began rattling off various incidents.

Any staff member in the Alzheimer's disease care facility would, I believe, tell you there was no real concern for their safety or for the safety of residents. Most would tell you how much they enjoyed being around Jo and how much they liked her and what a special lady she was.

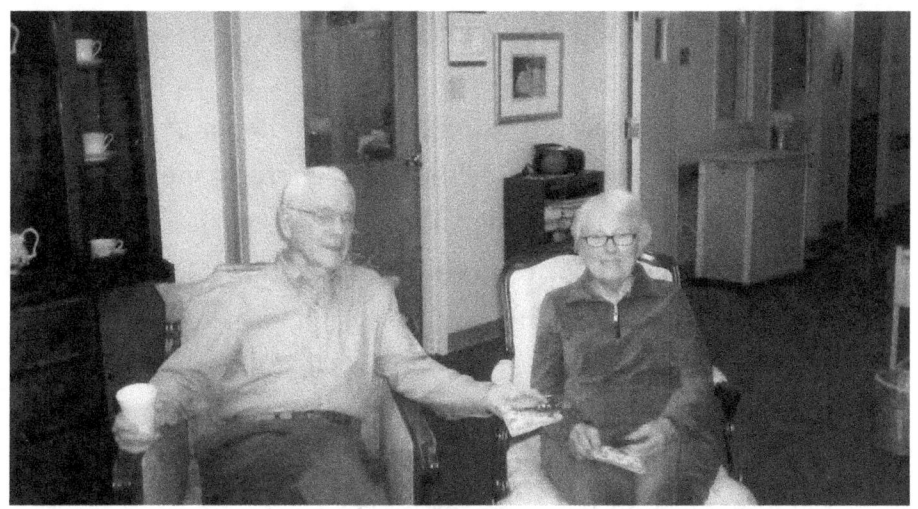

Claude and Jo Freeman, 2005

While Jo was a resident in the ALP/D facility, we would walk the hallways of buildings on campus. We knew how many laps to walk in the basement downstairs, then go up to the ground level where we would walk in the hallways the number of laps we needed to get the distance we intended to walk, before returning Jo to the ALP/D facility for the night. One night as we were walking, not talking too much, rather silently, Jo said "I hope someone in heaven knows your name."

As I sit here on February 18, 2011, writing *Jo's Story* I reflect on my daily written chronology of events from mid September 2005 to October 30, 2010.

After May 9, 2006, Jo perceived, sensed, knew there were new people involved in her care and the care of other ALP/D residents in the facility. Jo sensed the new persons involved then in her care were not friendly to her, they were not making an attempt to get to know her, or to make and be friends, they were irritating her by their actions, and perhaps their communications, causing an unpleasant atmosphere, which was tense and frightening.

Jo perceived accurately from May 9, 2006 her environment had changed drastically after she became aware of the presence of the new, unknown, unfriendly persons who created an atmosphere in which she became apprehensive, and fearful of.

Jo was perceptive of the care or lack of care, and the unfriendly persons assuming her care after May 9, 2006.

It became apparent to me during the summer and early fall of 2006 the ALD and Supervior of Staff at the ALP/D facility (SAS) could cause notice to be served on Jo and myself that Jo could or would be transferred from the ALP/D facility to assisted living on campus where there was no CCDI facility. I had observed former residents placed in the assisted living downstairs and I did not want Jo to become a resident there. There was no activity there and those former residents became mummified, sitting in a wheelchair or a recliner in front of a television set the greater portion of the day and gaining weight rapidly.

I did not want our alternative options for housing in the future to be limited to that.

During the year of 2006 I learned how very important the ability to communicate with Alzheimer's diseased persons is, and how equally important is hands-on care to which the Alzheimer's diseased resident is receptive and favorably responsive to. Those are two very important skills that direct care workers must have to be effective in their employment in a care facility where Alzheimer's diseased persons are residents.

The success as a caregiver and their relationship with an Alzheimer's diseased person is dependent upon communication skills and hands-on care to which the Alzheimer's diseased person is receptive of and favorably responsive to.

July 11, 2006

The next day I telephoned the neurologist and made an appointment for Jo. I also made an appointment with Jo's personal physician that morning. The next night, while sitting in the hallway downstairs after a walk, Jo asked me if she caused trouble for me. I responded that I didn't think she had. I didn't inquire further, but I wondered where that thought process came from, as I had never mentioned to Jo any of the complained-of events to evoke that thought process. My thought process at the time was that unless things were improved or changed in the scheduling of staff at the care facility, newly prescribed medication would not change Jo's reaction to boredom, inactivity, or having the feeling that she and others were being treated like third-graders.

The communications I had with the RN from June 30, 2006 through July 10, 2006, and especially the conduct of, and the remarks the ALD made, and then threats the ALD made on July 10, 2006, caused me to have great concern. Instinctively, after the July 10, 2006 meeting, I knew the procedure the ALD had implemented, her decisions, her strategy, her personal conduct, and her personal threats were not how an experienced, learned ALD employed in a certified ALP/D facility would proceed if a staff person informed that experienced, learned ALD it was perceived a resident in that ALP/D facility had a change of behavior. Even an inexperienced, untrained ALD, as a courtesy, would have discussed with the spouse of the ALP/D resident the perceived change in behavior before calling that resident's personal physician, reporting the perceived change of behavior, and requesting medication to treat the perceived behavior change.

Those experiences caused great dismay.

As I was reflecting today, February 18, 2011, I must have felt that the SAS and RN would realize there had been no change in Jo's behavior, and cause ALD to inform me to cancel appointments with the neurologist and Jo's personal physician, and come to the conclusion special medication was not required. The neurologist, as well as Jo's personal physicians, upon reflection, were of the opinion no medication was needed for the perceived aggressive behavior; seemingly to pacify ALD they prescribed Seroquel, low dose, for hallucinations, and both inquired of me if it was possible to place Jo at a different care facility.

I then gave serious thought as to our alternatives, and determined to do research concerning the prescribed procedure to address, do an analysis, and make an assessment of an Alzheimer's diseased resident's perceived change of behavior.

Commencing July 16, 2006 daily experiences limited my time to then obtain answers I wanted. Later I found the answers to many questions I then had, some of which you will find in this segment of *Jo's Story*. Other specific, detailed answers you will read in my Alzheimer's Disease paper located in the next segment of this book.

July 16, 2006

The following Sunday staff on duty failed to look at a note that had been left the night before by the 11 p.m.-7 a.m. staff. The note informed the morning shift that Jo had new pants to wear to church that day and that she should eat her breakfast in her robe, as recently cereal or juice had been spilled on her clothing she was to wear for an outing. That note was left but the 7-3 staff did not look at the note.

When I arrived at the care facility I observed Jo sitting at the breakfast table with her eyes closed. Before her was a piece of coffee cake from which a bite had been taken. Jo had a fork in her hand and there was something in her mouth, which she had not swallowed. I asked if she had eaten anything before getting the coffee cake and was informed she had eaten cereal. She had been given her medicine. Jo would not talk but was trying to make me understand, with her mouth full, that something was wrong. She would not swallow or take juice. Jo was very docile during this entire period of time.

Finally, she indicated she wanted to get rid of what was in her mouth. I held a napkin for her but liquid went through my fingers. I requested that the staff person get me a napkin and a towel. After clearing Jo's mouth, I took her to her apartment where she wanted to lie down on the bed. I determined immediately why Jo was acting as described above. The person who got her out of bed and assisted in putting her robe on failed to have Jo put her partial denture in her mouth. She was fed cereal, given her medication, water and/or juice, and staff did not notice her denture was not in her mouth.

It was my belief that Jo became aware that the partial denture was not in her mouth when she endeavored to eat the coffee cake. Jo is very sensitive about her teeth. I can understand her consternation when she realized the denture was not in her mouth.

I called staff to a place in the hallway near the kitchen and showed them the denture still in the nighttime container. At which time staff said they were sorry and apologized. Needless to say, we did not get to attend church wearing the new pants. That night staff on duty between 3 and 11 p.m. confirmed they observed the note that was left for the 7 a.m.-3 p.m. staff.

July 19, 2006

The following Wednesday, I requested the 3-11 p.m. staff leave a note for the staff scheduled to be on duty the next morning. The note was to say that the staff should get Jo up, dress her, feed her, and give her medication before 8:25 a.m., as I would be there at that time to leave for the 9:00 a.m. appointment with Jo's personal physician.

The next morning I received a phone call from the staff that Jo was up but would not take her medication and at the time had her partial denture in. I inquired who was on duty with her, and when I was informed who that person was, I suggested that person and Jo got along well and suggested that person could get Jo to take her medication.

The staff person then told me that person was not licensed to give medication. I suggested the staff person could stand by or position herself so that she observed the procedure. That staff person said she would think about it, but she wasn't so sure. I advised that staff person that I would be right over.

When I arrived, Jo had taken the medication, but was still sitting at the breakfast table. Jo was quite distraught. When she heard my voice she got up from her chair and hugged me very desperately. It was obvious to me that Jo had been subjected to something that really disturbed her. I tried to comfort her, reassure her, but did not really get her to respond favorably. I finally sat her in my lap at the table.

The RN and SAS were advised. It was determined I should take Jo to the Iowa Methodist ER, which I did. We never had an opportunity to talk to the doctor at the ER, but very competent people interviewed us, and tests, including a CT scan, were done. All tests were reported to be negative and normal. We then returned to the care facility. The next morning I called Jo's personal physician's office to inquire if the physician wanted me to bring Jo in and inquired if the faxed reports (from ER) were received by the office. They confirmed that the reports were received. Jo's personal physician did not request to see Jo. I then inquired as to when Jo could next see her doctor. I was advised the doctor would be gone for a week or so and the earliest appointment would be approximately one month later, which appointment was made.

August 2, 2006

It was now approximately one month since I was advised someone on staff had formed the opinion that Jo was a threat to safety of staff and residents. I knew that RN who previously reported to me aggression by Jo had recently, for a period of time, personally been around Jo with some regularity. Therefore I stopped to see her and inquire if there was a change in the thinking of the person who initially demanded a medical doctor prescribe for Jo a medication to control her alleged agitation or irritation, and to inquire if it was necessary for Jo to be seen by a neurologist for those reasons. That nurse informed me, in substance, that Jo should keep the appointment.

August 3, 2006

I received a call around 3:00 p.m. or so that Jo had fallen

and injured her arm. I went to the care facility and found various staff with Jo and I observed a prominence on her left forearm just above the thumb, with swelling and slight discoloration.

It was determined that an outside x-ray service should come to the care facility and x-ray the arm, which was done. The outside technician took the x-rays to a radiologist to review the films. We had to wait a period of time before the radiologist called to report there was a non-displaced fracture at the distal end of the radius of the left arm.

In the meantime someone called Jo's personal physician's office where a person gave permission to commence Tylenol 500mg every six hours for pain from the fracture.

Ultimately, arrangements were made for Fraser ambulance service to transport Jo and I to the Iowa Methodist ER for examination and treatment. It was very busy there and we waited a long time until a room was available, then, after we were placed in a room we were briefly interviewed, and informed we would have to wait for the caster. That person did not arrive until 10:45-11:00 p.m. After that the ambulance service was called and we returned to the care facility around 12:20 a.m. the next morning.

August 4, 2006

In the late afternoon of the next day I observed the back of Jo's left hand and thumb were swollen and very discolored and painful. The following morning the arm was very painful and discolored, not withstanding that ice packs that had been applied periodically as I suggested. Even the ice was painful. It was later suggested that ice be applied for only about 20 minutes per session.

The following day we did not go to church and Jo remained in pajamas and slept most of the day. I applied lotion and very gently massaged Jo's fingers and thumb. A nurse from the downstairs care facility cut the gauze from around the thumb where it was too tight and painful.

August 8, 2006

Two days later staff assisted Jo via wheelchair from the care facility to my car for the appointment with the neurologist scheduled for 11:20 a.m. Upon our arrival it was necessary for the use of the valet service. The neurologist, commenting after consultation and examination concluded, in substance, there was no need to prescribe medication for agitation. He did conclude he would communicate with Jo's personal physician and would suggest that after her scheduled appointment with Jo that she prescribe a very low dose, perhaps 20 mg, for hallucinations. The neurologist looked at Jo's left arm cast and discoloration of hand and fingers too. The neurologist inquired if it was possible to place Jo in a different Alzheimer facility, to which inquiry I responded, "No."

August 9, 2006

The neurologist apparently called Jo's personal physician concerning the cast and her hand condition, as the next morning the ALP/D nurse called to advise me that a person from Jo's personal physician's office called to inform that Jo's personal physician had made an appointment for her to see an orthopedist at 2:30 p.m. The nurse wanted to confirm that I could have Jo there for that appointment.

Jo and I drove out to the location of Jo's personal physician and the location of the orthopedist office complex. I parked very close to the entrance thinking Jo and I could easily walk that distance. I parked and walked around the car to assist Jo from the car, and as we were standing outside the car, as I was about to close the passenger door, Jo just sagged, or wilted downward. I caught her and raised her to a standing position, then asked her if she wanted to sit down in the car for a moment. She said no, she was alright. I then, while holding onto her, locked the door. No sooner than I had locked the door, she wilted or sagged again.

Fortunately, a lady saw the events and came to our assistance. The two of us got the car door open and sat Jo down in the car. Jo at no time came in contact with the surface of the parking lot as I was able to keep her from completely falling. The nice lady proceeded to the entrance to inform the valet of the experience as I was driving from the parking to the entrance for valet service. The valet service evidently passed on the information about our experience.

We arrived at the orthopedist office and found the nice lady from the parking lot there for a scheduled appointment too. A person came to the waiting room site and took information from both of us concerning the parking incident.

X-rays were taken while waiting and then the orthopedist examined Jo's cast and arm and concluded they would remove the original cast and apply a new cast, which would be slightly different and more manageable. The cast was pink, a color that suited Jo. The doctor requested and scheduled that we return in four weeks for a follow-up exam and change in cast.

August 18, 2006

Nine days later we appeared at Jo's personal physician's office. Her doctor began to inquire concerning matters the assisted living nurse and her director had previously communicated to that doctor's office. Jo was very aware of the conversation, in fact, at one point Jo interjected that I should allow her doctor to finish the question before I responded. The doctor silently smiled and raised eyebrows! Jo's doctor stated at the conclusion of the appointment the doctor would confer with the neurologist and then decide if medication would be prescribed for Jo's hallucinations. Jo's personal physician also inquired if there was a possibility that Jo could be moved to a different Alzheimer's care center. Later, at the conclusion of our appointment or meeting, and after hearing my answers to the doctor's questions, Jo, who had been sitting quietly said, in a very loud voice, as the doctor was leaving the room, "help he is going to kill me..."

By this time we were in the office hallway and a nurse on staff showed us to an unoccupied room where I talked with Jo. I endeavored to explain to her why we were there, and that I was merely answering the doctor's questions about complaints being made about her behavior. After assuring Jo everything was okay we left the office to proceed to the parking area. As we were departing from the parking lot Jo requested that I go straight to the river where we could "dump him" in the river.

I am not sure Jo remembered the alleged contentions asserted by staff from the care facility, therefore Jo must have perceived that I was making up stories to tell her personal physician, as Jo said later she "could never believe me again."

Jo continued the remainder of the day to be quite wary of me, but by evening consented to me assisting her in getting ready for bed and doing her dental hygiene.

These experiences for Jo and I were brought about by staff persons from the ALP/D care facility who filed reports of instances without investigating or knowing or understanding why a particular incident occurred. There was no urgent need for those staff persons to aggressively and forcefully push for medication to curb Jo's alleged agitation or irritation. Neither staff nor residents were at risk as they contended.

August 22, 2006

Four days later Jo's personal physician ordered 25 mg of Seroquel, one pill daily, which was given at 8:00 p.m. Seroquel is a very unpredictable medication, which, in my opinion, was not needed.

September 13, 2006

Staff had been advised for some period of time that Jo's cast was to be removed on September 13 by the orthopedist at 9:15 a.m. I had advised the staff we would leave for the appointment about 8:40 a.m. I arrived at the care facility and Jo was not dressed at 8:30 a.m., and she was a bit owly. I got her dressed, but she was very lethargic and apprehensive for some reason. We had talked for several days about how nice it would be to get the cast off. When we got into the car to depart for the doctor's office I placed the care facilities' forms on the console. As we were driving from the care facility Jo took that envelope in which the forms had been placed and would not give it back until the receptionist received it at the doctor's office. Jo feared I was going to take away more of her freedom.

It came time for us to go into the exam room, first to remove the cast and then for x-rays. The doctor's young assistant picked up the small electric saw and was demonstrating the procedure for removing the cast. But when she turned the saw on and Jo heard the noise and perceived the spinning blade, Jo became quite excited. It was then determined we would do the x-ray first, which confirmed a healed fracture.

The orthopedist then endeavored to coax Jo into removal of the cast but was not successful. The orthopedist then very kindly rescheduled us to come back to the office two days later to remove the cast.

September 13, 2006

Jo and I appeared at 1:15 p.m. at her ear, nose, and throat doctor's office without incident for her six-month appointment to check her ears for wax or for cleaning, during which the doctor found her ears to be clear but suggested we commence using prescribed eye medication on Monday and Friday nights, one drop in each eye.

September 14, 2006

Jo would not let the CNA dress her. Upon my arrival at Jo's residence at about 10:00 a.m., I was advised Jo had not taken her medications; those medications were given to me as I arrived. I had a bit of a hard time convincing Jo that she should take the medications, as Jo was very frightful, very anxious, and somewhat fearful of her surroundings. After taking her medications, she then allowed the CNA to dress her. After making certain that

Jo was comfortably resting, I left her place of residence contemplating my alternatives, as I was absolutely certain the Seroquel was affecting Jo adversely. I decided to personally communicate with Jo's physician requesting Seroquel be discontinued.

September 14, 2006

I faxed the following to Jo's personal physician: *Subsequent to Jo being seen by the neurologist you suggested on August 8, and seeing you August 18, it was determined that 25 mg of Seroquel would be prescribed for Jo.*

Jo has been given one 25 mg Seroquel tablet at approximately 8 p.m. each night for approximately three weeks. There has been a noticeable change in my wife.

The Seroquel was to control hallucinations, as I understood, to some extent. The hallucinations are rather constant presently. Jo has been having more frequent balance problems since she commenced taking Seroquel. She seems to be drowsy more frequently, and Staff have difficulty in the mornings getting her up out of bed, getting her shower, getting her dressed for the day.

I believe she is aware she is different for some reason, and she is not trusting of me or Staff at times, therefore the strange or different feeling frustrates her greatly, and causes her to become obstinate and confused. I undress her and get her dressed for bed, then assist her with her dental hygiene each night, but the last 10-14 days our usual pleasant procedure has become a tedious procedure.

It is my belief that we should discontinue the Seroquel for a period of time. Staff reported to me this morning that Jo was anxious, that she had breakfast, but would not let Staff assist her in dressing for the day, that she had been seen pushing a resident's walker, and that she had someone's sweater on. I arrived at the facility and found Jo had shoes and socks on, plus her pedal pusher pants, but still had her p.j. top on. Her partial denture was still in the container in which it was placed last night, and I was informed Jo had refused to take her Lexapro, Namenda, and Razadyne at breakfast. After much coaxing I was able to get her to take her medication, but she was very wary asking me several times what other problems I would cause for her, and inquiring of me how could I place her in this Class-B environment?

I do not want my relationship with my wife to be changed by a medication so unpredictable as Seroquel. Please give serious thought to discontinuing Seroquel for a period of time.

Thank you for your consideration.

Sincerely, Claude Freeman

Jo's personal physician, after receiving the above faxed correspondence, ordered on Friday, September 15, 2006, Seroquel be discontinued.

September 15, 2006

From September 13 to the morning of September 15 the care facility staff and residents talked to Jo about how nice it would be to have her cast removed on Friday. In fact, when I arrived at the care facility on the morning of the 15th, there appeared on Jo's door a drawing and writing announcing that Jo's cast would be removed that day, and several drawings of Jo's pink cast by a staff member whom I thanked. Jo was given a medication at 10:00 a.m. prescribed by the orthopedist or by Jo's personal physician for pain and/or to alleviate anxiety. Jo was in great spirits; she was seemingly her natural self. There was no fear, she was ready for the cast to be removed. She did not flinch one time during the procedure. And upon our return to the care facility the residents were just commencing their noon meal and as we entered the residents and staff all gave Jo a good welcome and hooray for the removal of the cast.

September 18, 2006

Monday, September 18, 2006, about 4:00 p.m. Jo and I were sitting on a loveseat in the main hallway when a friend on campus walked up and then sat down to visit. During which visit another person came and stopped by. The first friend turned and inquired of the second friend who stopped by if he took notes during the Campus Administrator's Monday Update or if anything new was discussed. This second person who stopped by said about the only thing he could recall was that the lady in charge of assisted living was leaving.

The next day the wife of a male resident of the same ALP/D facility where Jo was a resident had scheduled a birthday party for her husband, which was really nice. ALD attended the birthday celebration along with other residents and staff. During that celebration ALD appeared and assisted in serving the ice cream and cake and in doing so talked to several residents including Jo. During which, in exchange of greeting, Jo said to ALD, "I thought you were going, or leaving." The ALD answered, in substance, "No, I am not going." I presumed Jo recalled the remarks made the previous day when we were sitting on the loveseat visiting with the two people who had stopped.

The ALD left in October, 2006, I am certain, as November 6, 2006, the campus update publication announced the name of the new ALD.

The care facility in which Jo was a resident could accommodate nineteen residents. Ordinarily, between the hours of 6:30 a.m. and 11:00 p.m. there were only two staff persons on duty for nineteen residents. That two-person staff was made up of a nurse or a CMA and one CNA. Mid-morning a person acting as activity director would appear for a period of time and then depart; and at noon lunch a third person would generally appear to assist in serving lunch and assist for a period of time in which the residents were consuming or being fed their noon-time lunch.

During the afternoon there might be a third person present for a period of time also. From 3 p.m. to 11 p.m. most generally there were only two people, a nurse or a CMA and one CNA, on duty during those hours.

The staff-to-resident ratio of two staff to nineteen residents was not good. Various sources suggest the ratio should be at least one-to-five, that is, one staff person to five residents.

There were three persons primarily involved in this fiasco: the Supervisor of ALP/D Staff (SAS), the Assisted Living Director (ALD), and the RN.

The ALD commenced her position on Campus March 15, 2006; the RN had been in the Health Center on campus before her current assignment; I do not know with any certainty when the SAS came on board. I did not recall seeing the RN in and around the ALP/D facility too frequently after October. The SAS remained in and around the facility, and at times endeavored to be friendly, but read her communication directed to me later regarding Seroquel along those lines.

I never learned, and do not know now, the education of the SAS, or of her training or experience in the care of Alzheimer's diseased persons. Through my observations of the SAS's care of a resident and listening to her communications in her effort of the care of a resident would cause me to believe the SAS had little or none.

I would be certain the SAS began to inform the ALD of incidents attributed to Jo. The content of this communication caused the ALD, who had been on the job only four months, to overreact; both on the couple of occasions that I observed where she publicly expressed herself, and the manner in which she directed the RN and/or the SAS to proceed. Initially, calling the office of Jo's personal physician, the communications with persons therein, communications related to the Executive Director of the campus, her actions and public conversation, and her invitation to Jo to go to the courtyard, then not meeting and taking Jo into the courtyard as the ALD suggested—these all are indicators of how insensitive the ALD could be in communicating with and caring for the need of one Alzheimer's diseased resident and her family.

I visited several times with the RN and related to her as indicated in this writing my thoughts. If the RN communicated those thoughts to the ALD and or the SAS, they gave no credence or consideration to my logical thinking and explanations as to their perceived changes in Jo subsequent to Jo being informed her newfound friend had made her decision to further her education, and leave ALP/D.

The experiences Jo and I had in the ALP/D facility between July and October 2006 caused me to dig deeply to learn more about Alzheimer's disease, and care procedures advocated, for residents in facilities that are certified to care for Alzheimer's diseased residents therein, especially as the Alzheimer's disease of those resident's progresses.

In June and early July, without proper prescribed analysis and assessment it was wrong for one or two staff persons to label Jo as a problem, then to telephone Jo's personal physician requesting medication be prescribed for problems those staff persons perceived. Those persons persisted in labeling Jo as a problem not withstanding the comments and observations I made to the nurses.

In my "Alzheimer's Disease Paper," a part of this publication, I refer to a 2006 publication by Elizabeth C. Brawley, *Design Innovations for Aging and Alzheimer's*. Brawley points out: "There are seniors who are bored, helpless, and lonely in facilities all over the country. This means we urgently need to move beyond the medical model of care and embrace a more social model that focuses on the individual in a meaningful, life-affirming way." Further, Brawley discloses: "Studies have shown that the environment strongly influences behavior, particularly the behavior of those with Alzheimer's disease and related dementia… Communication is the cornerstone of nonpharmacological treatment in habilitation therapy, which is radically different from traditional forms of therapy for older adults…. Caregivers are expected to change their own behavior or change the environment rather than expecting the person with Alzheimer's to change. This is undoubtedly a more accountable approach with a much higher rate of success."

October 19, 2006

October 19, 2006, I arrived at the care facility and Jo was napping. The SAS followed me into Jo's room and informed me that Jo had been sad, that she had been talking about her mother, then the SAS had patted Jo and Jo had reached up to hug the SAS and thanked her.

I had a different reaction, however, as I heard that person's remarks made in Jo's presence. Nonetheless, on this occasion, that conversation, intended for my information and heard by Jo, didn't have an adverse reaction by Jo.

October 20, 2006

Subsequently, on a day I returned from the supermarket, I noticed someone had called and left a message for me to come to the ALP/D facility as soon as possible. I put my groceries away and went to the care facility, arriving there at approximately 11:00 a.m. where I was met by the SAS who informed me that Jo did not want to get up when a staff member went in to wake her, and did not want to take her regular morning shower.

I went into Jo's room as the SAS was telling me the above and I began talking with Jo who appeared very weary at 11:00 a.m. I went out to determine if Jo had been given her medication and was informed that she had not. It was then some eighteen hours since she had had her last medication at 5:00 p.m. the previous day. It had been approximately 24-26 hours since she had been given Lexapro, which is prescribed to be given once a day, usually at breakfast. The two other medications, Razadyne and Namenda, are usually given at breakfast and at dinner, or the suggested twelve hours apart.

I asked for and was given the three medications, I poured a

cup of apple juice and went to Jo's room where she took without resistance the pills and drank all the juice. I then talked Jo into taking a shower and dressing if the one CNA who usually bathed Jo was then available. That CNA agreed and came to Jo's room to get Jo and her clothes. Jo was then a bit hesitant or reluctant. I noticed Jo did not have her denture in, so I had her put her denture in and then brushed her teeth before walking into the shower room where the CNA had gone to prepare her clothes and bath.

Jo was still a bit apprehensive once we were in the shower room but with the CNA's patience, Jo was showered and dressed. During the time Jo was in the shower room the SAS thanked me for coming. She then preceded to tell me that earlier they had Jo coming into the dining area to eat, but she didn't want to eat, or wouldn't sit down to eat. She said that while Jo was in the dining area she grabbed or jerked the walker of one of the other residents and did a similar movement of the walker of another resident. The SAS tried to impress upon me some sort of aggression on Jo's part, contending the residents were just eating their breakfast and had not done anything to aggravate Jo.

The SAS related that when the Seroquel was discontinued it was suggested that Jo be seen again by neuro-psych or a neurologist. She then talked about an annual conference with staff members regarding Jo.

I suggested that perhaps it was the environment causing Jo those frustrations. I then inquired if the SAS had seen rubber gloves scattered on the floor of Jo's room, taken from a box of gloves that had been left on a shelf above the coat hanger rod just outside Jo's bathroom. Or if she had noticed the small wicker basket on the floor in which band aids and small wooden dental picks and other items had been but were now on the floor by the table next to Jo's bed. I said the strewn items would suggest that Jo had problems this morning getting things done and couldn't independently get done.

It was obvious that certain staff had not been trained to make valid analysis and assessments of Alzheimer's diseased resident's actions or conduct.

After showering and dressing it was then time for lunch; I sat Jo down for lunch at a table with two other residents, put an apron on Jo, then went into Jo's room where I waited until Jo finished her lunch. Staff informed me that Jo ate all of her lunch, after which she took a nap.

Jo and I took a walk later in the afternoon and before I left about 4:00 p.m., I informed the 3-11 p.m. staff that Jo did not take her three medications until 11:15 a.m., therefore only about six hours would have passed when staff would ordinarily give her two medications at 5:00 p.m.

It was decided that those medications would not be given until around 8:00 p.m., hoping the next three would be given by 8:00 a.m. the next day. After I had my dinner I returned to the care facility. Jo and I went for a walk, then did our nighttime regular routine, during which time the 3-11 p.m. staff came in and gave Jo her two medications and put prescribed eye drops in her eyes.

October 31, 2006

Jo was scheduled for a dental appointment at 2:00 p.m., of which staff had been advised. When I arrived to get Jo she was not completely dressed. I began to assist her, and then suggested we brush her teeth at which time I noticed the partial denture was not in place. I went to talk with the SAS about that fact and on the way back to Jo's room the SAS began telling me all the food Jo had eaten. She then left and returned with the CNA, who was new to me. The CNA advised me she had put in Jo's denture earlier that morning, and did not know now why the denture was at this time in the pink container lying in water; I suggested we talk about it later, not in Jo's presence. It was then about 1:35 p.m. I was thinking as the CNA talked, if the denture had been in Jo's mouth earlier, who actually took it out and put it in the pink box, put water in the box and then put the detached lid securely on the box? Why wasn't Jo dressed at 1:35 p.m. as I had suggested previously? How many times has staff failed to have Jo ready to depart for an appointment when previously informed of the appointment and suggested time of departure?

November 24, 2006

On November 24, 2006, I was enroute to Jo's place of residence at about 2:50 p.m. As I arrived at the elevator the 3-11 p.m. CMA arrived at the same time. We rode the elevator together to the ALP/D facility. Upon my arrival I found Jo lying on her bed, partially covered by a blanket, one leg and foot was not covered and I noticed the pant leg was blue, not the green pants I had laid out the night before. No shoe was on her stocking foot and I noticed a stain on the stocking. Her bra was on the floor, green shirt on the chaise, shoes on the floor, bathroom light was on, odor in bathroom with toilet filled with bowel movement.

I then noticed the green pants lying on top of the wire basket-type cabinet. The pants were badly soiled, her panties were in trash basket, badly soiled. I immediately called the CMA and the CNA to observe and survey the situation, which was then about 2:55 or 3:00 p.m. We uncovered Jo to begin the cleanup and observed she had no bra on, no panties, the blue pants she had on were soiled since she had not wiped good before putting them on.

Taking into consideration the things observed and assuming Jo received no help from the 7 a.m.-3 p.m. staff, all this would have taken place over a period of at least 45 minutes before the 3-11 p.m. CMA and I arrived in the care facility. Where was the 7 a.m.-3 p.m. staff for those 45 minutes? The 3-11 p.m. CNA had arrived a few minutes before me and the CMA. It was obvious Jo could not get to the bathroom in time to get her pants down and get seated on the stool in time. She did ultimately get them down and get seated as there was considerable bowel movement in the stool, unflushed. After finishing her bowel movement, I presume she took her shoes off, pulled her green pants off, pulled her panties off, and was appalled by the experience. She obviously felt all her clothes were dirty and she needed a shower, as she removed her shirt and bra too. She then went to her closet and found the blue pants to put on. Too humiliated and in a sense of futility, she just covered up and hoped a friend would find her and help her. What an experience.

November 28, 2006

As I entered the ALP/D facility and began to walk down the hall I observed the SAS walking toward me carrying a red collarless pullover type shirt on a hanger, with Jo in tow and another ALP/D resident in tow. The SAS appeared to me as if the SAS was an elementary school teacher with two third graders in hand was taking them to their room or to the office for a good talking to! I just reached out for Jo's hand, which Jo gave me, then I took Jo to her room, without any words said. The SAS never mentioned the event subsequently. Again, the SAS's method of dealing with the situation did not suggest to me the SAS knew anything about problem solving in an Alzheimer's facility.

Jo perceived accurately, from May 9, 2006, her environment had changed drastically after she became aware of the presence of the new, unknown, unfriendly persons, especially the SAS who created an atmosphere in which Jo became apprehensive, and fearful of.

Because of the varied experiences Jo had in the ALP/D facility, especially subsequent to 5-09-06, I endeavored to learn more about the written, publicly advocated care of Alzheimer's diseased residents in care facilities. Persons at the Alzheimer's Association Greater Iowa Chapter called to my attention a publication from the Alzheimer's Disease and related Disorders Association, Inc. in 1997 entitled *Key Elements of Demenia Care* (hereinafter referred to as KEOD 1997). I was also advised that a 2006 book entitled *Mayo Clinic Guide to Alzheimer's Disease* would provide reliable information about diagnosis, treatment, and caregiving for Alzheimer's disease and other forms of dementia. In addition, my attention was directed to Elizabeth C. Brawley's book *Design Innovations for Aging and Alzheimer's: Creating Caring Environments*, all of which I quote and make reference to in my "Alzheimer's Disease Paper" signed 1-12-07.

I have learned that the "old styled institutionalized care method" is not good, nor is the understaffed, untrained care givers tendency to heavily sedate or place in restraints an Alzheimer's diseased person. There is a movement toward humanized care, with a new conceptual model for care of the frail elderly and chronically ill. This radical new approach to long-term care refines and redesigns how care is delivered to elders in an environment that promotes independence, dignity, privacy, and choice.

In the 1997 publicaton *Key Elements of Dementia Care*, it is pointed out that Alzheimer's/dementia care is unique and ever-changing. "Persons with dementia and their families have unique needs; programs, environments and care approaches must reflect this uniqueness. As the field of Alzheimer's/dementia care continues to evolve so must our efforts to provide the best quality of care." (Page 5)

In this publication, providers are encouraged to explore their commitment and grow to become "dementia-capable." "Dementia-capable means skilled in working with people with dementia and their caregivers, knowledgeable about the kinds of services that may help them, and aware of which agencies and individuals provide such services. This means being able to serve people with dementia, even when service is being provided to other people as well. Dementia-specific, on the other hand, means that services are provided specifically for people with dementia."

It is suggested (page 11): "Developing an effective care/service plan for a person with dementia requires careful assessment of that person...and attention to the unique features of dementia."

In a section entitled "Problem Analysis and Resolution" (page 16) it is suggested: "Address difficult behaviors analytically, (e.g., leaving the care setting, or entering unsafe places or rooms of others, repetitively asking questions, striking other people or disrobing.) Assessment of the individual in the situation which the behaviors are occurring is important... <u>Analysis of the behavior and its causes should precede any consideration of use of medication or physical restraints to control behavior.</u> Table 2 outlines a simple problem solving method of resolving challenging behavior)." (Emphasis supplied)

The following are excerpts from Table 2 (page 17) in the section "Problem Analysis and Resolution" in *Key Elements of Dementia Care*:

Table 2: Problem Solving Outline for Challenging Behavior

Assess the Behavior to Discern Why the Resident Is Engaging in the Behavior

1. **Describe in detail the behavior.** Include what occurs, when it occurs, how often it occurs, and who else tends to be involved in the situation in order to discern the pattern of the behavior... Describe conditions regarding the behavior. Identify what preceded and what resulted from the behavior...

2. **Examine the extent to which the behavior is a problem.** Identify <u>who is raising the concern about the behavior</u> (family member, caregiving staff, the person with dementia, or other residents). <u>Who experiences the behavior as a problem?</u> Is anyone in physical or other danger as a result of the behavior?...

3. **Try to discern why the resident is engaging in the behavior by examining 1 and 2 above.** ...Did something in the environment trigger or cause the behavior? For example,

is there too much, too little, or an inappropriate type of stimulation? Is there a change in the environment?...

(Underlined emphasis supplied.)

Continuing in "Problem Analysis and Resolution" (page 18) it is further noted that "Staff caregivers could easily over-react or react in a counterproductive way to certain behaviors, if assessment is inadequate... Choosing an intervention from among the options brainstormed is greatly facilitated by thorough assessment. Trial and error can be costly and time consuming, as well as potentially harmful to the person. If the behavior and its conditions, the individual's wishes and needs, and the genuine requirements of the caregiving setting are all adequately assessed, many 'difficult' behaviors can be fairly easily resolved, while still maintaining the individual's dignity, comfort, and pleasure."

"The degree of success in assessment and care planning depends upon the extent to which the assessment and care planning are individualized and flexible, so they can adapt to small and major changes over time. Blanket or corporate care plans designed to have the person fit the program rather than the program adapt to the individual are the least successful. If a person no longer 'benefits the program,' then the program should change to fit the person, rather than the person be discharged."

Under "Staffing Issues" in the same book (page 48), it is noted that "Not everyone is personally suited to work with persons who have dementia. The ability to operate effectively in a context in which roles are flexible and the focus is person-oriented instead of task-oriented is not universal. The ability to enjoy working under such circumstances should be identified among the requirements for employment in this field."

Under "Recruitment and Hiring" (pps. 52-53) in the same book: "Recruiting caregiving staff who reflect the qualities needed to provide dementia-capable care is definitely a learned skill. Working with dementia residents requires specific attributes and skills that go beyond a generic care program. Job descriptions and individual performance goals should include the values articulated in the program philosophy and mission statement."

"Select caregiving staff for the special care program based on their experiences and commitment to the unique demands of caring for someone with dementia. Being successful in another area of the setting does not mean the individual is appropriate for the dementia care program. Find out if staff members want to work with residents with dementia. Before transferring staff to a dementia program, be sure the staff views the transfer as a reward for their hard work as opposed to punishment."

In the 2006 book entitled *Mayo Clinic Guide to Alzheimer's Disease*, in a section entitled "Strategies for Behavioral Symptoms," wherein it is reported: "Challenging behaviors often associated with Alzheimer's include:

- Aggression
- Agitation
- Delusions
- Hallucinations
- Resisting Help
- Suspiciousness or paranoia
- Sleep disturbances
- Wandering

"It's important to remember that someone with Alzheimer's is gradually losing his or her language skills and ability to communicate. These behaviors may be the only way that person can express discomfort, stress and frustration."

On page 104, it is pointed out: "Without much thought it would be easy to label a challenging behavior, or even the person with Alzheimer's who displays that behavior, as 'bad' or a 'problem.' It's important to resist labeling for two reasons. For one thing, troublesome behaviors are rarely acted out on purpose or manipulatively—they arise from the disease process. For another thing, these labels create the expectation that there is 'good' behavior—an expectation that the person might not be able to meet. Unfilled expectations may foster a sense of futility, resignation or anger."

Strategies that may help in dealing with behaviors are referenced on pages 104-107, to which strategies I now allude:

"Many times behavioral problems occur not because of cognitive impairment but because of secondary issues. Health, psychological, environment and social factors all can have a profound effect on a person with dementia."

"**Environmental factors**. Understimulation or overstimulation within a person's surroundings can have a significant impact on his or her behavior. With nothing to do, a person with Alzheimer's may become bored or restless and resort to wandering or yelling to release frustration... Creating a safe, serene and predictable environment can provide a sense of familiarity and comfort for the person with Alzheimer's and reduce the risk of disruptive behavior.

"**Stay engaged.** One way to improve quality of life and prevent challenging behaviors from developing is to make sure the person with Alzheimer's is involved with daily activities and routine tasks. Staying occupied can make the person feel that he or she is needed and participating in the normal rhythms of life."

It was rather ironic to me that the neurologist that Jo was referred to inquired of Jo during our visit on August 8, 2006, and his examination of Jo, observing the cast on Jo's left arm, asked if it was possible to place Jo in a different Alzheimer's facility; to which inquiry I responded, "No."

Then subsequently at the August 18, 2006, appointment with Jo's personal physician, that physician also inquired if there was a possibility Jo could be moved to a different Alzheimer's care facility.

I had been informed in 2004 and 2005 the ALP/D facility in which Jo was placed was one of the best, if not the best, in Des Moines. I decided if this ALP/D facility was one of the best, why move her to a strange environment?

December 6, 2006

For some period time it was hot in the ALP/D facility resulting in dehydration of various residents. The heat at times was very oppressive.

At about 3:45 a.m. I went to Jo's room to check on the heat. Very hot, I opened the window. At 9:45 a.m. I discussed the oppressive conditions with various maintenance employees who related the equipment in the ALP/D facility was basically old equipment with automatic valves; the system was not functioning correctly, sending water running through the pipes at 210 degrees.

That night it was very hot again and I requested that a security person come and turn off the radiator in Jo's room. The pipes and the turn-off valve in that radiator were so hot they burned the security person's hand, who then needed a bath towel to turn the valve off.

Old antiquated equipment, bad for residents.

December 20, 2006

It was determined Jo had a kidney infection, and the doctor prescribed and ordered Bacitrim, an antibiotic, which Jo was to take for seven days. Jo took the last dose at 8:00 p.m. on December 26th.

January 4, 2007

The CMA on duty from 3-11 p.m. telephoned me to inform me that while eating supper Jo had to go to the toilet to have a bowel movement. Jo went to the toilet located in the dining area near where Jo had been seated. Jo was in the toilet alone and while there she did not get seated on the toilet or did not get her clothes down in time, or for some reason made a mess on the floor of the toilet.

The CMA checked on her after a while and found Jo trying to clean the area where a mess had been made in the toilet room. It was a bad experience, I was informed by the CMA. Again, only two staff persons were on duty at the time for nineteen residents.

January 7, 2007

No church. After breakfast I was assisting Jo from the table to her room, and as we neared her doorway, she wilted. We got Jo into a chair and slid her into her room. Very scary, as there were then no responses by Jo.

The CNA and I tried to get Jo to respond, but none. The CNA called for the nurse from downstairs to come and check. We finally got Jo to open her eyes and to respond to a degree. It was determined she should be taken by ambulance to the Iowa Methodist ER where IV fluids were given and we saw a rapid change in awareness. She had a low blood pressure reading but all other tests were normal, but for dehydration.

We returned to the care facility, ate lunch saved for her, asleep by 2:00 p.m., long nap, but was thirsty by 4:00 p.m. Given more water, perked up and ate supper. She slept between 6:00 p.m. and 7:00 p.m.

January 10, 2007

Jo fell in her room; no apparent injuries. Several residents had the flu. CMA came in to work as usual around 3:00 p.m. She said she had become ill about 1:30, but no one was available to substitute for her. She remained on duty until after supper.

January 15, 2007

I received a call from the RN in the a.m. that Jo had fallen, but there was no apparent injury. Unfortunately, I had a touch of the flu or something, which caused a rather severe case of vomiting. That same day I received a second call around 5:00 p.m. from the RN that Jo had fallen again, in her room, with no apparent injury except a laceration on her right forearm. I was quite concerned, but did not dare go to the facility as I was not sure whether I had the flu or food poisoning.

January 17, 2007

I was feeling better and felt that I could go to Jo's care

facility without infecting anyone. Jo and I walked around the area several times and I noticed no serious problems. I went back and visited again in the afternoon and walked Jo and noticed no changes or signs of injury, except that at times she would close her eyes. I went back over after dinner and while getting her ready for bed, I found she had pain when attempting to rise and stand erect. The pain seemed to be in the right hip area.

January 18, 2007

I arrived at Jo's care facility about 7:00 a.m. and had a discussion with the CMA regarding Jo's falls and pain complaints. I requested that when the RN came in at 9:00 a.m. that the CMA and RN telephone the office of the orthopedic person who re-casted Jo's arm and make arrangements for Jo to be taken by a care facility bus to that orthopedic office for x-rays to determine if previous falls had resulted in a fracture.

Upon my arrival at 1:00 p.m. at Jo's care facility I inquired about the status of things. Because of the flu and illness and absenteeism, it was suggested that I discuss Jo's condition with a substitute former employee. I did so and after talking to that person I went to Jo's care facility where I found Jo at a table in the dining room. That former employee was now feeding Jo a second cup of ice cream. Jo's eyes were closed, there was plate in front of her where there was a wet-looking croissant with tuna salad or some other ingredient. I also noted the pink container in which we put Jo's denture every night before putting her to bed. The lid was off the container sitting in front of Jo and the denture contained therein could be easily seen by two residents also seated at the table. Jo knew the denture was not in her mouth and I called that to the attention of the former employee and then suggested that we talk in the office after getting Jo to her room.

Apparently the former employee had not been advised of my request for x-rays. It was reported that the RN and the ALD had called in sick. After my visit with the former employee she called Iowa Methodist ER and an ambulance. Jo was examined, tested, and x-rayed and treated in the ER. She was admitted to the hospital late that night.

Jo's Alzheimer's disease had progressed further, and there were threats that Jo might be removed from the ALP/D facility to a nursing unit that was not a certified CCDI (Chronic Confusion Dementia Illness) unit.

On January 18, 2007, as Jo received care at Methodist Hospital, I contacted staff at a CCDI facility that had opened in October, 2006. The staff was very accommodating. On January 22, 2007, when Jo was released from the hospital, she was taken to and became a new resident at that CCDI facility where she remained until her death at 7:02 p.m. on October 30, 2010.

The majority of the staff at the ALP/D care facility were very nice, kind, pleasant staff persons. After researching the prescribed, advocated procedure to be followed by staff concerning a resident's perceived behavior change, it is my observation that one person who appeared to me to assume the position as supervisor of the staff at the ALP/D facility classified Jo as an agitator and a threat to staff. The SAS reported the same to the ALD, who was unqualified for the position and, because of her inexperience and lack of knowledge, had allowed herself to be drawn by her underling into strange territory in which she thought force and threats would alleviate a perceived problem, which never, in fact, ever existed.

Alzheimer's Paper

PREFACE

The loved one of the person writing this paper is an Alzheimer's diseased resident in an Iowa Alzheimer's/dementia care facility.

Since the loved one announced early one morning in Arizona, some six years ago, she had a problem, the two have attempted to deal with the then unknown problem, which problem was initially diagnosed as a benign memory loss, later as Alzheimer's disease.

The experiences the two have had with medically trained individuals, medicines prescribed by physicians, home caregiving, transfer of care to an Alzheimer's/dementia care facility, and experiences at that care facility, have caused the writer to seek knowledge concerning the diagnosis of Alzheimer's disease, the treatment of and the giving of care to Alzheimer's diseased persons.

Initially, it seemed information was rather sparse, then one day the writer ventured into the Alzheimer's/Organization Greater Iowa Chapter where he looked at printed materials on a bookshelf, and met Ann Riesenberg, RN, MA, CHPN, who visited briefly about Alzheimer's, and encouraged the writer to return at anytime he felt a need to discuss or inquire further about Alzheimer's or caregiving.

During the several years of being a home caregiver and later observing caregivers in a care facility, the writer continued his endeavor to seek information about caregiving to Alzheimer's diseased persons.

The writer became informed concerning the current prevalence of Alzheimer's, and it's predicted ascendency by year 2050.

The experiences the writer and the Alzheimer's diseased loved one have had, and the predictability that many other families and their loved ones will incur similar experiences, provoked and prodded this writer to publish this paper. It is his endeavor to cause an individual person, a neighborhood, city, county, state, and national awareness to Alzheimer's disease.

You will read in this paper of the prevalence of Alzheimer's. (Prevalence is defined: *the percentage of a population that is affected with a particular disease at a given time.*)

You will read that Alzheimer's disease is prevalent. (Prevalent is defined: *widespread, being in ascendency.*)

Because of it's prevalence and the predicted ascendency of Alzheimer's disease by 2050 it is imperative various educational institutions—including medical schools, governmental bodies, and including agencies, administrators of, owners of and providers of Alzheimer//Dementia care facilities, Alzheimer's/dementia care facility program directors and caregivers in Alzheimer's/dementia care facilities—need to be better informed, educated, trained, and experienced in caring for, and communicating with, in a type of an environment prescribed herein. (Imperative is defined: *an obligatory act or duty.*)

As one reads this paper you will learn that the "old-styled institutionalized care method" is not good, nor is the understaffed, untrained caregivers' tendency to heavily sedate or place in restraints an Alzheimer's diseased person.

You will read there is a movement toward humanized care, with a new conceptual model for care of the frail elderly and chronically ill—a radical new approach to long-term care that refines and redesigns how care is delivered to elders in an environment that promotes independence, dignity, privacy, and choice.

In this paper I endeavor to cause persons to become aware of the prevalence of Alzheimer's disease and its predicted ascendancy, and once those persons who read this paper become aware, motivate those persons to "make a difference" in the care given Alzheimer's diseased persons by creating premier Alzheimer's resident care facilities staffed by the best Alzheimer's disease educated and trained personnel in the State of Iowa.

Signed by Claude H. Freeman, 1-12-07

ALZHEIMER'S DISEASE

In a publication of Alzheimer's Association , Chicago, Illinois, entitled "One of Our Greatest Medical Challenges," it is reported in 2006 "Alzheimer's is a devastating disease that impairs memory, reasoning, motor skills and the ability to take care of oneself. The impact of Alzheimer's on individuals, families and our health care system makes the disease one of our nation's primary medical, social and fiscal challenges.

"Alzheimer's affects every level of our society, and the statistics associated with the disease are sobering:
* an estimated 4.5 million Americans have Alzheimer's disease
* by the year 2050, the number of Americans with Alzheimer's could skyrocket to 16 million
* half of adult Americans age 35 and older know someone with Alzheimer's disease
* one in 10 individuals over 65 and nearly half of those over 85 are at risk of the disease

"No one knows what causes Alzheimer's disease, but continued funding, unrelenting advocacy and dedicated individual efforts can help conquer it."

In that same Alzheimer's Association publication referenced above it is suggested "Consider, for example, that more than seven out of ten people with Alzheimer's disease live at home, where almost 75 percent of the care is provided by the family. The average lifetime cost of care for an individual with Alzheimer's is $174,000. A person with the disease will live an average of eight years and as many as 20 years." (Attachment A)

In *U.S. News & World Report* dated December 11, 2006 in the "Health & Medicine" section is an article entitled "Alzheimer's Today." At Page 74 the following is written: "Recently, thanks to better diagnostic tests that lead to earlier detection, the medical community has started to recognize that dementia is an equal-opportunity destroyer. 'In the last five years, more younger people have been showing up at support group meetings and in doctor's offices, asking for help, and we realized this is something we need to start taking seriously,' says neurologist Ronald Petersen, an Alzheimer's and memory disorders specialist at the Mayo Clinic. It afflicts people in their 50s, their 40s and even in their 30s. 'Alzheimer's is not just a disease that hits 80-year-olds in nursing homes,' says Dallas Anderson, a specialist in the epidemiology of dementia at the National Institute on Aging."

At page 76 of the "Alzheimer's Today" article the following appears: "To rule Alzheimer's in or out, a patient's family history is examined. That's especially important with early-onset victims, since a large number of them have a close relative who had serious memory problems. Then the patient undergoes a series of neuropsychological tests. 'We need to find memory impairment plus problems in at least one other domain, such as attention or language,' says David Salmon, a neuropsychologist and Alzheimer's specialist at the University of California-San Diego. If dementia is the likely suspect, brain scans such as magnetic resonance imaging or positron emission tomography can help zero in on the specific type. So can a spinal tap. 'None of these are good enough by themselves,' says Petersen. 'So you have to put them all together. Then you can look at your patient and say, "I hate to say it, but it looks likely to be Alzheimer's.""

And then you talk to them about medications like Aricept or Namenda, which seem to keep the disease at bay for awhile.'"

Would it be prudent to advocate, legislate, or require persons who reach a prescribed, specified age to be tested to determine those most likely to become an Alzheimer's diseased person?

Ann Riesenberg, RN, MA, CHPN, Program Director, Alzheimer's Association-Greater Iowa Chapter reported November 13, 2006, that there are currently approximately 68,000 Alzheimer's diseased persons living in Iowa. That 68,000 number is expected to rise or increase as the large number of so-called baby boomers reach ages referenced above.

I am advised the following are facilities in Iowa where care is given.

1. Assisted living: this setting is for residents who are somewhat independent; the resident has some infirmity which requires some assistance from staff; ordinarily no Alzheimer's diseased person would be a resident there.

2. ALP/D facility: this type of facility is defined below more specifically. It is a dementia specific program, a secured facility.

3. CCDI facility: this type of facility is defined below more specifically. It is a secured facility where Alzheimer's diseased residents in Stages 4, 5, and 6 are usually housed, where residents who have a tendency to wander are placed; residents who are combative are not placed herein, nor are addicts placed in a CCDI facility.

4. Nursing facility: resident is placed in such a facility when total care is needed.

5. Skilled nursing care: ordinarily no Alzheimer's diseased resident is transferred to skilled nursing for care.

It is reported in materials circulated in 2006 by the Alzheimer's Association-Greater Iowa Chapter that there are currently 37 ALP/D Programs-facilities (Dementia-specific assisted living programs—a program that serves five or more tenants with dementia between Stages 4 and 7 on the Global Deterioration Scale and hold itself out as providing specialized care for persons with dementia in a dedicated setting). The total capacity of those 37 ALP/D facilities =2273.

Those 37 ALP/D facilities are located in the nineteen counties listed below, and opposite each listed county you will find the number of ALP/D facilities located therein, plus the total resident capacity.

County	ALP/D Facility	Resident Capacity
Blackhawk	1	128
Buchanan	1	84
Cedar	1	70
Clay	1	111
Clayton	1	38
Clinton	1	44
Dubuque	1	104
Henry	2	84
Jackson	1	63
Johnson	2	84
Linn	6	428
Marshall	1	64
Polk	5	208
Pottawattamie	1	26
Poweshiek	1	52

County	ALP/D Facility	Resident Capacity
Scott	6	438
Wapello	1	133
Washington	1	10
Woodbury	2	104
19	37	2273

How aware is the State of Iowa that only nineteen Iowa Counties out of 99 Iowa Counties have ALP/D Programs (Dementia-specific assisted living programs—a program that serves five or more tenants with dementia between Stages 4 and 7 on the Global Deterioration Scale and hold itself out as providing specialized care for persons with dementia in a dedicated setting)?

It is also reported in materials circulated in 2007 by the Alzheimer's Association-Greater Iowa Chapter there are currently 116 CCDI facilities ("Chronic Confusion or Dementing Illness" is a special license classification for nursing facilities or a special unit within such a facility providing care to persons who suffer from chronic confusion or dementing illness. Reference to Chronic Confusion of Dementing Illness Units [CCDI] is made in the acts and joint resolutions of the 1990 regular session of the Seventy-Third General Assembly of the State of Iowa.) The total capacity of those 116 CCDI facilities = 2314.

Those 116 CCDI facilities are located in the 70 counties listed below, and opposite each listed county you will find the number of CCDI facilities located therein, plus the total resident capacity. It is to be noted the CCDI facilities are exclusively for Alzheimer's diseased residents.

County	CCDI#	Resident Capacity
Allamakee	2	20
Audubon	2	39
Benton	1	13
Blackhawk	2	54
Boone	2	56
Bremer	1	30
Buena Vista	1	20
Calhoun	1	10
Cass	1	24
Cedar	1	6
Cerro Gordo	3	41
Clarke	1	29
Clay	1	11
Clayton	1	16
Crawford	1	24
Dallas	3	59
Decatur	1	12
Delaware	1	16
Dickinson	1	14
Dubuque	2	28
Emmet	1	15
Fayette	2	24
Floyd	2	36
Franklin	1	19
Greene	1	10
Hamilton	1	15
Hancock	1	12
Hardin	2	32
Harrison	1	18
Howard	1	34

County	CCDI#	Resident Capacity
Humbolt	1	24
Ida	1	17
Jackson	1	37
Jasper	2	40
Jefferson	1	14
Johnson	1	25
Jones	1	24
Kossuth	1	14
Lee	4	80
Linn	5	120
Lyon	1	9
Madison	1	18
Marshall	2	96
Mitchell	1	14
Monona	1	20
Montgomery	2	28
Muscatine	1	19
O'Brien	2	30
Palo Alto	1	8
Plymouth	2	31
Polk	9	237
Pottawattamie	1	15
Poweshiek	1	16
Ringgold	1	8
Sac	1	12
Scott	5	167
Shelby	2	36
Story	2	48
Tama	3	42
Van Buren	1	18

County	CCDI#	Resident Capacity
Wapello	1	20
Warren	4	100
Washington	2	25
Wayne	1	13
Webster	1	30
Winnebago	1	14
Winneshiek	1	10
Woodbury	2	62
Worth	2	27
Wright	1	20
70	116	2314

How aware is the State of Iowa that only 70 Iowa counties out of 99 Iowa counties have CCDI facilities? ("Chronic Confusion or Dementing Illness" is a special license classification for nursing facilities or a special unit within such a facility providing care to persons who suffer from chronic confusion or dementing illness.)

Note: the 16 counties underlined are reported to have both ALP/D and CCDI facilities located therein. The three counties not underlined on the ALP/D report are Buchanan, Clinton, and Henry, therefore it is assumed they have no CCDI facility.

Counties not listed on the ALP/D or the CCDI reports are: Adair, Adams, Appanoose, Butler, Carroll, Cherokee, Chicksaw, Davis, Des Moines, Fremont, Grundy, Guthrie, Iowa, Keokuk, Louisa, Lucas, Mahaska, Marion, Mills, Monroe, Osceola, Page, Pocahontas, Sioux, Taylor, Union. Am I to presume these 26 counties have neither an ALP/D facility nor a CCDI facility?

54 of the 74 counties listed on the CCDI report are not listed on the ALP/D report. Am I to presume that any person in those counties diagnosed as being an Alzheimer's diseased person has no choice in that County other than to become a resident in the CCDI facility? Does this mean all Alzheimer's diseased persons in that county are consolidated or housed together in that CCDI facility?

80 counties out of 99 Iowa counties reportedly have no ALP/D facility, is that correct?

29 counties out of 99 Iowa counties have no CCDI facility, is that correct?

Who compiled the ALP/D and CCDI lists provided? I have been advised the Department of Inspections and Appeals compiled the list, and endeavors to update it daily.

What criteria was applied to compile the lists? I have been advised the Department of Inspections and Appeals staff apply pertinent Iowa Code sections to determine facilities that pass requirements specified that are regulated by that Department; those that meet the criteria specified are placed on the appropriate list.

What known facilities exist where Alzheimer's diseased persons reside that are not on these lists?

Why aren't those facilities on the lists? Or on a list indicating they have residents, but are not approved, or some indicator?

How can a facility be in operation to care for Alzheimer's diseased persons and not be on one of these two lists?

Do the Departments of Elder Affairs and Inspections and Appeals collaborate on the rules and regulations that determine, control, and affect care Alzheimer's diseased persons receive, or at times is there an imaginary, territorial, or departmental line not to be crossed?

Do treating physicians of their Alzheimer's diseased patients have any knowledge as to what an ALP/D or CCDI facility is?

In the event all 68,000 Iowa Alzheimer's diseased persons sought residency in an Iowa ALP/D facility or CCDI facility, their endeavor would be futile, as the listed ALP/D facilities capacity is 2,273 persons, and the listed CCDI facilities capacity is 2,314 persons, for a total capacity of 4,587 persons. Assuming that 75% (51,000) of the 68,000 Alzheimer's diseased Iowans live at home, as suggested in the Alzheimer's Association publication referenced above. In the event 4,587 are actually residents in the above-listed ALP/D and CCDI facilities, where do the remaining 12,413 Alzheimer's diseased receive care prescribed for their diseased condition?

How concerned, interested, and informed are the people in Iowa about Alzheimer's disease?

How concerned, interested, and informed are the people in Iowa about persons in Iowa who have Alzheimer's disease?

Persons generally do not become concerned, interested, and

informed about matters unless and until we or our loved ones are affected by a condition or an event. When we or a loved one are diagnosed as having Alzheimer's disease we then become quite concerned, very interested, and endeavor to become well-informed about Alzheimer's disease, including the prescribed treatment, care, environment, and then we endeavor to learn how the quality of the life of the Alzheimer's diseased person can be extended until the fatality of the disease occurs.

Let us conclude more than 37 ALP/D Program-facilities and the 116 CCDI facilities listed above are presently needed, and in the future more such facilities will be needed for Alzheimer's diseased Iowans.

Who will pay for, design, construct, furnish, staff, manage, and oversee those ALP/D and CCDI facilities?

Alzheimer's facilities must conform to present-day criteria prescribed for the care of Alzheimer's diseased residents!

What are the design criteria for a current day, efficient, effective Alzheimer's care facility?

How are an Alzheimer's diseased resident's needs to be met and provided in current day Alzheimer's disease care facilities?

We learn after much reading, personal interaction, observation, and discussion an Alzheimer's diseased person's quality of life can be extended in the proper environment, staffed with persons educated and then trained to interact, communicate, and accurately assess each individual Alzheimer's diseased resident's needs in that environment, where there is an effective Activity Program in which all staff members and all Alzheimer's diseased residents are involved and participate.

ALZHEIMER'S CARE FACILITY

Elizabeth C. Brawley, IIDA, AAHID, President of Design Concepts Unlimited , a San Francisco-based firm that specializes in designing living environments for older people and settings for Alzheimer's special care caused to be published in 2006 a book she wrote entitled *Design Innovations for Aging and Alzheimer's* (herein after referred to as Brawley's 2006). Brawley is a past member of the national board of directors for the Alzheimer's Association and has gained international recognition as an expert and industry leader in the area of environmental design for aging. She is also the author of *Designing for Alzheimer's Disease: Strategies for Creating Better Care Environments* (Wiley), which was awarded the Joel Polsky Prize by the American Society of Interior Designers in recognition of her outstanding contribution in the area of research in environment and Alzheimer's disease.

In the preface of Brawley's 2006 book one will find when reading the same, excerpts such as:

> Studies suggest an important element of successful aging is a person's ability to age in place in a stable living environment.

> While care is part of the package when needed, the focus is on living.

> Guided by a philosophy of caring, the term *life-enhancing environment* describes the physical and cultural atmosphere created to support older residents. The major environmental

factors influencing physical health and emotional well-being are sound, light, and sense of touch. The significance of the physical environment increases if judgment and mental competence fade.

Studies have shown that the environment strongly influences behavior, particularly the behavior of those with Alzheimer's disease and related dementias.

Activity should be the heart of long-term care and is an area that needs and deserves open minds, open communication, and cooperative planning between design professionals and healthcare providers to create the very best caring environment.

The mistake that most often hampers the planning process is having no strong activity program and waiting to hire an activity director after the building is complete. This strategy has proved only moderately successful at best.

Brawley points out in her 2006 book in Chapter 3 entitled "Environment as Treatment" on Page 28, "The new emphasis on nonpharmacological treatments and our growing understanding of neuroscience is sparking the imagination of caregivers, clinicians, designers, and others concerned with people living with dementia."

In Brawley's 2006 book at Page 32: "Special care settings, from adult day care to assisted living to nursing homes, that face major renovation or new construction should carefully consider the value of designing rather than decorating or making constant 'quick fixes' to these environments. When the increase in quality of life and the potential decrease in medication costs are weighed, it may turn out that making environmental changes will pay off."

Brawley discloses in her 2006 book on Page 34, "Communication is the cornerstone of nonpharmacological treatment in habilitation therapy, which is radically different from traditional forms of therapy for older adults. Accepting the frame of reference and definition of 'reality' of the person with dementia is an essential part of this communication, as is the premise that actions speak louder than words in order to change behavior. Caregivers are expected to change their own behavior or change the environment rather than expecting the person with Alzheimer's to change. This is undoubtedly a more accountable approach with a much higher rate of success."

"What Is Culture Change?" is the title of Chapter 11 in Brawley's 2006 book. Commencing at Page 147 Brawley relates: "Culture change is a continuing process of growth." It is reported that "culture change is the new buzzword in long-term care." Nursing home culture change means systemic change throughout a facility from both the individual and the organizational perspective... The goal is creating a culture of aging that is life affirming, satisfying, humane, and meaningful."

At page 148 Brawley points out "there are seniors who are bored, helpless, and lonely in facilities all over the country. This means we urgently need to move beyond the medical model of care and embrace a more social model that focuses on the individual in a meaningful, life-affirming way."

In Brawley's 2006 at Page 168 Brawley points out that "older residents need a sense of control over their lives and environment, the freedom to discover others and enjoy life— especially at a time when decisions are too frequently made for them."

In discussing resident bedrooms Brawley relates at Page 182, "In a shared environment, private rooms provide one space that can be shaped to the individual's personal taste and made uniquely his or her own. They help give residents a sense of control over their environment in a setting where opportunities for this are often limited."

Chapter 15 at Page 223-224 in Brawley's 2006 is entitled "The Green House." It is reported there, "Astoundingly a typical resident in a nursing home receives only 70 minutes of care per day, five minutes from licensed nursing personnel and the remainder from the certified nursing assistant."

Brawley points out that the philosophical foundation of the Green House Project is drawn from the work of Dr. William Thomas, MD. "...a movement toward humanized care, with a new conceptual model for care of the frail elderly and chronically ill—a radically new approach to long-term care that redefines and redesigns how care is delivered to elders.

"The Green House places the primary focus on the elder's quality of life... The goal of this new model is to provide frail elders with an environment that promotes independence, dignity, privacy, and choice."

At Page 152 Brawley points out that "Long-term care becomes an environment for meeting resident needs rather than institutional needs." It is pointed out by Brawley that culture change in long-term care must start at the top through governance and the executives, permeating every part of the organization. There is no cookie-cutter approach, and it will never happen if the whole organization is not involved.

Does culture change work? Brawley reports at Page 158 that "in a three-year study recently completed in New York state,

culture change was shown to have substantial beneficial conse-
quences for residents and staff. Resident health and well-being
was enhanced, relationship building between staff and residents
increased. There was increased social activity, less depression,
and a reduction in falls, weight loss, and dehydration."

The following is taken from Brawley's 2006 book, Chapter 20,
entitled "What Does Success Look Like and How Will You
Know?"

> Successful settings truly focus on their residents and design
> and build environments that support their philosophy of care.
>
> Success doesn't start with the physical environment. While it's
> easy to fall in love with a beautiful building, it's not always as
> easy to fit the program into the structure. Too many projects
> are built only to make caregivers struggle to mold programs to
> fit the building. Designing the activity program comes before
> the building design. The architectural design responds to and
> accommodates the program–the activity spaces, workspaces,
> and the variety of therapeutic, recreational, and social needs
> as well as living accommodations of residents and staff. The
> design for the physical environment is based on meeting pro-
> gram needs. Identifying, describing, organizing, and designing
> the varied and often complex activity-based programs to be
> included can begin before the architectural design team is on
> the scene.
>
> It is still important to make a clear distinction between the
> programs and needs (recreational and therapeutic activities)
> defined by the staff and the program describing spaces and
> space adjacencies referenced by architects and designers.
> Because the same word (program) is used to refer to these
> very different concepts, those involved in planning often hear
> very different things based on their areas of expertise and
> may make questionable decisions if they misunderstand the

context. Make the distinction, make the distinction again, and continue to clarify the use of the word *program* to eliminate confusion and ensure the success of the design for all parties–planners and users.

The best projects start by defining goals, articulating what's important, and looking at the organizational and staffing components. Then comes the hard work of figuring out how to maximize the way the building can support your goals. Providers must be clear in conveying to architects how they want particular features to work and what results they expect to achieve. When there is a clear understanding of the project goals it is far easier to achieve good design solutions. This step may take some time. A lot of hard work must be done before the pencil is put to paper designing. This step also provides the foundation for post-occupancy evaluation.

For current design criteria, based upon Brawley's personal family experience with Alzheimer's disease and personal memory loss resulting from radiation and chemotherapy for colon cancer, Brawley's professional experiences, achievements, and professional recognition, one would highly recommend to organizations or persons who are interested in or who are contemplating constructing, improving or remodeling an Alzheimer's/dementia care facility they refer to, adopt, apply, and use criteria set forth and advocated in Brawley's 2006 book *Design Innovations for Aging And Alzheimer's.*

What is the philosophy of the State of Iowa concerning current existing Alzheimer's/dementia care facilities and their certification?

What new or different criteria will the State of Iowa enact, establish and require before it will in the future certify Alzheimer's/dementia care facilities because of culture change in long term care?

MISSION STATEMENT

In a book published by Alzheimer's Disease and Related Disorders Association, Inc. in 1997 entitled *Key Elements of Dementia Care* (hereinafter referred to as KEOD 1997) Section 1 thereof is entitled "Alzheimer's/dementia Care Focus." In the Introduction it is pointed out that "Alzheimer's/dementia care is unique and ever-changing. Persons with dementia and their families have unique needs; programs, environments and care approaches must reflect this uniqueness. As the field of Alzheimer's/dementia care continues to evolve so must our efforts to provide the best quality of care." Providers are encouraged to explore their commitment and grow to become "Dementia-Capable."

What do we mean by "dementia-capable"?

In KEOD 1997, Section 1, Page 5 it is defined as follows: "Dementia-capable means skilled in working with people with dementia and their caregivers, knowledgeable about the kinds of services that may help them, and aware of which agencies and individuals provide such services. This means being able to serve people with dementia, even when service is being provided to other people as well. Dementia-specific, on the other hand, means that services are provided specifically for people with dementia."

(Continuing, Section 1, Page 5) "Care settings can become dementia-capable only if individual staff members within the setting are also willing to become dementia-capable... Making a decision to become 'dementia-capable' includes examining the following:

* What does commitment mean to you and your care setting?

* Are you committed to putting philosophy into practice? What do these practices look like?

* How much can you realistically undertake and are you willing to do?

* Are you willing to make necessary changes?

* Will you identify indicators for improvement?

* Will you encourage open communication (i.e. family/resident councils, staff support programs)?"

It is pointed out in the KEOD 1997 publication that every care setting should have its own mission statement, which mission statement "drives the setting and includes the philosophy and how it will be implemented... The mission statement of a specialized Alzheimer's/dementia care program or setting should include the following:

* Program philosophy;

* Who the program serves;

* The approach to care;

* How and by whom care will be provided;

* The program location; and

* What is 'special' about the Alzheimer's/dementia care provided."

In KEOD 1997, Section 1, Page 6 it is pointed out that "the

program philosophy is a fundamental component of the mission statement. The program philosophy:

* describes the purpose and intent of Alzheimer's/dementia care

* recognizes the unique needs of persons with dementia

* is the basis or foundation of the program

* is supported by adequate resources

* is reinforced by policies and procedures

* has the commitment of all staff including direct care staff, managers, administrators, governing bodies, and owners

* is made operational by staff

"Who the program serves identifies the target population and is clarified in the policies, and discusses limitations of program, who can't be served, and reasons for transfer or discharge.

"The approach to care should disclose the intended approach to:

* physical, psychosocial, spiritual and emotional needs

* medical care needs are routinely assessed and met

* care/service plans are developed and implemented

* change in condition is recognized and addressed

* quality care is provided"

HOW AND BY WHOM CARE WILL BE PROVIDED, THE PROGRAM LOCATION, AND WHAT IS SPECIAL ABOUT CARE PROVIDED are found in KEOD 1997 and can be easily referenced there.

It is pointed out on Page 10 of Section 1 KEOD 1997 that "maintaining your commitment to provide dementia-capable care takes time, hard work, and most significantly, dedication. Since Alzheimer's/dementia care is continually evolving, providers must be dedicated to providing opportunities for ongoing staff education and training. At the same time, necessary changes or adaptations must be made to the care setting or program, after careful monitoring and evaluation."

What is the philosophy and mission statement of the care facility in which your loved one is an Alzheimer's diseased resident?

ALZHEIMER'S CARE FACILITY STAFF AND CAREGIVERS

It is my understanding the Iowa Department of Inspections and Appeal, upon approval, issues to a care facility a two-year Certificate, and at the end of the two-year period there is an inspection before there is a renewal of the Certificate.

What are the requirements that must be met before the initial certificate is issued?

Before a new Certificate is issued at the end of the two-year period what is the inspection criteria before another two-year recertification is made or given?

Are the inspection records before certification, and subsequent inspection records, conformance, or lack of conformance records available for public review?

Assume there are 68,000 Alzheimer's diseased persons currently living in Iowa, and further assume 75% (51,000) live at home, and assume the remaining 17,000 are residents in some form of an assisted living environment.

Records disclose 2,273 could reside in the 37 ALP/D facilities referenced herein. If we assume those facilities adhere to the 1:5 staff-to-resident ratio those combined facilities would need between them 455 staff persons, which staff would be there only for their eight-hour shift.

Records disclose 2,314 could reside in the 116 CCDI units referenced herein. If we assume those facilities adhere to the 1:5 staff-to-resident ratio those combined facilities would need between them 463 staff persons, which staff would be there only for their eight-hour shift.

Where do the remaining 12,413 Iowa Alzheimer's diseased persons receive care prescribed for their diseased condition?

Are each of the facilities in which those 12,413 Alzheimer's diseased persons reside certified as an Alzheimer's/dementia facility?

Specific staff-to-resident ratios have not been established, but in 1987 the Office of Technology Assessment suggested 1:6 for special dementia programs. Based upon focus groups conducted with experienced dementia caregiving staff, the ideal recommendation was a ratio of 1:5. Some authorities suggest that late afternoon and early evening when resident's energy level wanes, becomes tired, and after dinner becomes less energetic, and ultimately needs assistance getting ready for bed, there should be a higher staff ratio to resident ratio, perhaps a ratio of 1:4.

In the September 2006 Alzheimer's Association publication

entitled "Campaign for Quality Residential Care" (hereinafter referred to as: Alz Assoc 2006) at Page 7 it is recommended or suggested "staffing patterns should ensure that residents with dementia have sufficient assistance to complete their health and personal care routines and to participate in the daily life of the residence."

If the facilities in which those 12,413 Iowa Alzheimer's diseased persons adhere to the 1:5 staff-to-resident ratio there would be a need for 2,483 staff persons, which staff would be there for only their eight-hour shift.

Should the 1.5 staff-to-resident ratio be implemented for more than eight hours? If so, there would be a greater need for staff persons.

The facility must have adequate staff on duty at all times to be aware of and tend to the needs of residents as they spontaneously arise at all times of the day or night.

It is requested by this writer the staff-to-resident ratio between 8 a.m. and 8 p.m. be 1:4 in an Alzheimer's/dementia Care Facility.

Some dementia-specific providers have found it helpful to rotate staff periodically to prevent burnout.

What will or can be done to motivate and cause more capable, young persons to become interested in Alzheimer's/dementia care as an avocation?

What specific education and training must an Alzheimer's staff person receive before becoming employed as a staff person in an Alzheimer's care facility?

What practical experience must a staff person have before actually becoming employed and having personal contact and responsibility with and for an Alzheimer's resident in a unit or program such as an ALP/D facility?

Attached hereto are copies 321-25.34(231C) Dementia-specific education for program personnel, and 58.54(6) re: staff working in a CCDI unit or facility. (Attachments B and C)

Do treating physicians, of their Alzheimer's diseased patients, have any knowledge of what education, training, experience, or certification caregivers in ALP/D or CCDI have? Should the treating physician have some knowledge as to who his Alzheimer's diseased patient's care is entrusted?

What knowledge do the physicians, of their Alzheimer's diseased patients, have concerning the environment in which their Alzheimer's diseased patient is a resident?

What credence should the treating physicians give to reports called in to their offices from an ALP/D or CCDI care facility re: the care of the physician's patient—a resident then in an ALP/D or CCDI facility, especially if a prescription to sedate or a request for restraints is made?

What school or educational setting is licensed or authorized to educate prospective Alzheimer's caregivers ?

Are the educators, presenters, or trainers required to be certified or licensed before they endeavor to educate persons seeking to become or be educated as contemplated in the two attachments referenced above and attached hereto?

The environment, activity, or lack thereof, and staff in a facility in which Alzheimer's diseased persons reside greatly affect the life and behavior of that Alzheimer's diseased person.

In Alz Assoc 2006 at Pages 13-14 it is reported that "frequent, meaningful activities are preferable to a few, isolated programs. Activities should proactively engage residents. Design interactions to do with—not to or for—the resident. Every event, encounter or exchange between residents and staff is a potential activity. Dining is a meaningful opportunity for socialization, enjoyment, satisfaction and self-fulfillment. It is also pointed out that social engagement of residents is not the sole responsibility of the activities staff. Every staff member has the responsibility and the opportunity to interact with each resident in a manner that meets the resident's needs and desires.

"There must be daily activities, including Saturday and Sunday, residents must be kept active, residents must stay engaged. Residents are dependent upon the program director or activities director and staff to keep them involved in activities.

"The facility must have a knowledgeable, experienced, and stimulating program director or activities director."

Does the facility where your Alzheimer's diseased loved one is a resident have a knowledgeable, experienced, and stimulating program director or activities director?

Is each and every resident therein a regular, active participant in the activities?

In KEOD 1997, SECTION V, Page 51 entitled "Human Resources," it pointed out that "the caregiving staff has to provide continuity in care; residents need to feel safe and comfortable, and families need to be able to relate to and trust the caregiving staff."

"Both residents and their families rely on caregiving staff for:

* Compassion and concern for persons with dementia, their families, as well as for one another

* Respect and honor for the life lived by the person with dementia and his/her need to maintain continuity on living that life

* Helping the resident and family members adjust to the setting and maintain the highest levels of well-being and independence possible

* Creativity and innovation in finding solutions to sometimes complex care questions

* Dependability in maintaining a comfortable and understandable social environment

* Flexibility in providing all aspects of care and milieu (environment, surroundings) management

* Fairness toward persons with dementia whose behavior is sometimes difficult to understand

* Enabling persons with dementia to do as much as they can for as long as they can

* Sensitivity to diversity among persons with dementia, families, and co-workers

* Honesty in acknowledging what we 'don't know' as caregivers

* Integrity in providing services that are personalized and meaningful to persons with dementia

* Loyalty to underlying values that guide day-to-day care practices

* Appreciation of mutuality, or give and take between themselves and residents

* Patience, perseverance, and humor in assisting, facilitating, and supporting persons with diseases to achieve and maintain optimal function

* Supportive, caring attitudes and methods that are communicated to resident and family

* Appreciation of teamwork as a vehicle by which high quality, compassionate care is provided to persons with dementia"

(Taken from the Alzheimer's Association ACE Philosophy Training Program, Handout 1.10)

On Page 48 of KEOD 1997 under "Staffing Issues" it is noted that "not everyone is personally suited to work with persons who have dementia. The ability to operate effectively in a context in which roles are flexible and the focus is person-oriented instead of task-oriented is not universal. The ability to enjoy working under such circumstances should be identified among the requirements for employment in this field."

"Recruitment and Hiring" is a topic in KEOD 1997 at Pages 52-53. "Recruiting caregiving staff who reflect the qualities needed to provide dementia-capable care is definitely a learned skill. Working with dementia residents requires specific attributes and skills that go beyond a generic care program. Job descriptions and individual performance goals should include the values articulated in the program philosophy and mission statement."

Page 52: "Select caregiving staff for the special care program based on their experiences and commitment to the unique demands of caring for someone with dementia. Being successful in another area of the setting does not mean the individual is appropriate for the dementia care program. Find out if staff members want to work with residents with dementia. Before transferring staff to a dementia program, be sure the staff views the transfer as reward for their hard work as opposed to a punishment."

When there is an opening or a need at the Alzheimer's/dementia care facility where your Alzheimer's diseased loved one is a resident, and a need arises to hire or replace a director of assisted living, an RN, or other staff therein, what individuals or entities conduct the search to locate qualified persons for the required or vacated positions?

For the vacated or newly designated position or positions what credentials are required and specified?

Once prospects are located, who at or from the Alzheimer's/dementia care facility then personally interviews the prospective staff persons?

Who at or from the Alzheimer's/dementia care facility actually hires the prospective staff person or persons?

Recruiting caregiving staff who reflect the qualities needed to provide dementia-capable care is definitely a learned skill.
—KEOD 1997

Does the person or persons who do the recruiting, interviewing and hiring at the Alzheimer's/dementia care facility where your Alzheimer's diseased loved one is a resident have that learned skill?

What is the accurate, valid accreditation or certification of each staff person assigned to the Alzheimer's/dementia care facility where your loved one is an Alzheimer's diseased resident?

Is there a law or a departmental requirement that the current accurate, valid accreditation or certification of staff persons assigned to an Alzheimer's/dementia care facility be on display?

It is suggested in the KEOD 1997 book at Page 11, "Developing an effective care/service plan for a person with dementia requires careful assessment of that person, a detailed plan, and attention to the unique features of dementia."

Are the treating physicians of their Alzheimer's diseased patients familiar with the assessment practices advocated in KEOD 1997 and the Mayo Clinic Guide to Alzheimer's Disease?

On Page 16 of the above referenced publication a section is entitled "Problem Analysis And Resolution" wherein it is suggested:

> Address difficult behaviors analytically, (e.g., leaving the care setting, or entering unsafe places or rooms of others, repetitively asking questions, striking other people or disrobing). Assessment of the individual in the situation in which the behaviors are occurring is important.
>
> Analysis of the behavior and its causes should precede any consideration of the use of medication or physical restraints to

control behavior. (Table 2 on Page 17 outlines a simple problem solving method of resolving challenging behavior.) (Emphasis supplied)

In that book, on Page 17, there is Table 2-Problem-Solving Outline For Challenging Behavior, wherein it is suggested, among other things:

Table 2: Problem Solving Outline for Challenging Behavior

Assess the Behavior to Discern Why the Resident Is Engaging in the Behavior

1. Describe in detail the behavior. Include what occurs, when it occurs, how often it occurs, and who else tends to be involved in the situation in order to discern the pattern of the behavior... Describe conditions regarding the behavior. Identify what preceded and what resulted from the behvior...

2. Examine the extent to which the behavior is a problem. Identify who is raising the concern about the behavior (family member, caregiving staff, the person with dementia, or other residents). Who experiences the behavior as a problem? Is anyone in physical or other danger as a result of the behavior?...

3. Try to discern why the resident is engaging in the behavior by examining 1 and 2 above. ...Did something in the environment trigger or cause the behavior? For example, is there too much, too little, or an inappropriate type of stimulation? Is there a change in the environment?...

(Underlined emphasis supplied.)

Continuing on Page 18 of Problem Analysis and Resolution it is further noted that staff caregivers could easily overreact or react in a counterproductive way to certain behaviors, if assessment is inadequate. [See page page 74 in *Jo's Story* where that subject is addressed.]

In order to make a valid assessment, a staff person must be trained and experienced, must be intent on accurately determining the cause of the behavior, knowing well the resident, and truly endeavor to determine if the environment or a change in the environment, or activity, or lack of activity is cause of the behavior.

Nothing is more devastating to an Alzheimer's diseased resident and spouse than for staff to improperly and incorrectly assess the resident, report their assessment to resident's personal physician, which results in the physician prescribing a highly unpredictable medication.

Has staff personnel at the facility where your Alzheimer's diseased loved one is a resident been educated and trained in the prescribed assessments procedures advocated in KEOD 1997 and in the *Mayo Clinic Guide to Alzheimer's Disease*?

Does staff at the facility where your Alzheimer's diseased loved one is a resident follow the prescribed assessment procedures advocated in KEOD 1997 and the *Mayo Clinic Guide To Alzheimer's Disease*?

DEHYDRATION

In the *Mayo Clinic Guide To Alzheimer's Disease* at Page 319 there is the topic entitled "Dehydration." It is reported there that "people with dementia may forget to drink enough fluids. Signs of dehydration include dry mouth, little or no urination, weakness, dizziness or lightheadedness. Dehydration also can increase confusion and cause constipation, fever and a rapid pulse."

Room temperatures that are constantly too warm, 77 degrees and hotter, especially during night time, when Alzheimer's diseased residents are sleeping, can greatly affect hydration, causing a resident to become dehydrated during the 8-12 hours the resident remains in bed or in the confines of the resident's bedroom at those hot temperatures.

It is imperative that staff in the care facility be able to regulate temperature in the facility at all times. Too frequently maintenance personnel assume that control, which is ill advised, especially on weekends. In some care facilities maintenance personnel set a computer on Friday afternoon to control temperature in the facility from Friday through Sunday night, which causes serious problems for staff and residents if the temperature in the care facility is constantly 77 degrees or hotter over that extended period of time.

Usually old, antiquated boilers, furnaces, and a lack of functional thermostatic controls are the cause or causes of the problems alluded to herein.

DISPENSING MEDICATIONS

It is noted that an RN and LPN may dispense medications to residents in an assisted living care facility, and that a CMA may dispense certain prescribed medications to residents therein.

What academic courses, teaching, or training does a CMA receive before the CMA actually commences dispensing to Alzheimer's diseased residents medications prescribed by their personal physicians for the Alzheimer's diseased resident?

Some medications may be prescribed to be given to the resident 10-12 hours between doses, or prescribed to be given or taken with food or a breakfast and dinner (supper).

If medication is to be given or taken with food or at breakfast and dinner (supper) is a CMA instructed or trained to wait for all residents in the Alzheimer's diseased facility to be seated at their dining table for their meal, and during that dining experience, the CMA is to move from the medicine closet to the resident's place at the dining table and endeavor to cause that resident to swallow multiple prescribed medications prescribed for that resident, along with the consumption of a liquid presented to that resident, then proceed from the first resident to each and every other resident seated for dining, until each resident's prescribed medications have been dispensed to each resident, as each resident has been endeavoring to consume the food placed before the resident?

If a resident is distracted during meal time, being asked to then consume prescribed medications, sometimes with a mouthful of food, a resident may refuse the medications, or reluctantly take the medications, which may result in aggression, agitation, or somewhat resist help from the CMA, neither which is good for the resident endeavoring to enjoy the food placed before the resident for consumption.

Surely that CMA procedure would not be advocated by an instructor or teacher, one skilled or learned in Alzheimer's/dementia care.

What procedure(s) should or could be implemented to avoid such a distracting, dining room table, public dispensing of medications to Alzheimer diseased residents who are focusing on eating the food being placed before them for consumption?

Should there be implemented a procedure requiring the CMAs to dispense or give to each individual resident privately, in their private or individual room, before meals or after the time?

In the Alz Assoc 2006 publication at Pages 9-10 entitled "Adequate Food and Fluid Consumption" the following are suggestions, recommendations or goals:

> Residents should have a pleasant, familiar dining environment free of distractions to maximize their ability to eat and drink.
>
> To promote mealtimes as pleasant and enjoyable activities. Mealtime provides an opportunity for staff to observe and interact with residents, helping to ensure health, well-being and quality of life.
>
> To assure proper nutrition and hydration so that residents maintain their nutritional health and avoid unnecessary health complications, given resident preferences and life circumstances.
>
> Insufficient consumption or inappropriate food and fluid choices can contribute directly to a decline in a resident's health and well-being.
>
> Ongoing monitoring of residents is necessary to discover changes in food and liquid intake, functional ability or behaviors during meals. Any changes should be reported to dietetic staff and care planners.

I TRUST, AFTER READING THIS PAPER YOU WILL "MAKE A DIFFERENCE" IN THE CARE GIVEN TO ALZHEIMER'S DISEASED PERSONS?

Signed Claude H. Freeman, January 12, 2007.

ATTACHMENT A

Note: The reported $174,000 average lifetime cost of care for an individual with Alzheimers may be a bit low.

It is believed some ALPD facilities currently charge $100.00 - $125.00 per day; some CCDI facilities charge $185.00 - $220.00 per day per resident. The following figures are daily rates multiplied by 365 to arrive at the yearly costs.

$100.00 ($36,500.00); $125.00 ($45,625.00); $185.00 ($65,525.00); $220.00 ($80,300.00).

Note: When Jo was transferred to the CCDI facility in January 2007, it is my best recollection the daily rate was then $220.00. That daily rate was increased four times; the first yearly increase was $1,606, 2nd $3,285, 3rd $2,153.50, 4th effective 7-01-10 was $3,540.50, which increased the total by $10,585.00. Effective 7-01-10 the daily rate was $249.00 X 365 = $90,885 yearly rate, which was from January 2007, an increase of $10,585.00 in approximately 42 months.

ATTACHMENT B

Elder Affairs (321)
Chapter 25
Assisted living Programs
IAC 4/14/04

321–25.34(231c) Dementia-specific education for program personnel.

25/34(1) All personnel employed by or contracting with a dementia-specific program shall receive a minimum of six hours of dementia-specific education and training prior to or within 90 days of employment or the beginning date of the contract.

25.34(2) The dementia-specific education or training shall include, at a minimum, the following:

    a. An explanation of Alzheimer's disease and related disorders;

    b. The program's specialized dementia care philosophy and program;

    c. Skills for communicating with persons with dementia;

    d. Skills for communicating with family and friends of persons with dementia;

    e. An explanation of family issues such as role reversal, grief and loss, guilt, relinquishing the care-giving role, and family dynamics;

    f. The importance of planned and spontaneous activities;

    g. Skills in providing assistance with instrumental activities of daily living;

    h. The importance of the service plan and social history information;

    i. Skills in working with challenging tenants;

    j. Techniques for simplifying, cueing, and redirecting; and

    k. Staff support and stress reduction.

25.34(3) All personnel employed by or contracting with a dementia-specific program shall receive a minimum of two hours of dementia-specific continuing education annually. Direct-contact personnel shall receive a minimum of six hours of dementia-specific continuing education annually.

25.34(4) An employee who provides documentation of completion of a dementia-specific education or training program within the past 12 months shall be exempt from the education and training requirement of subrule 25.34(1).

ATTACHMENT C

Inspections and Appeals (481)
Chapter 58
Nursing Facilities
IAC 12/1/99

58.54(6) All staff working in a CCDI unit or facility shall have training appropriate to the needs of the residents. (II.III)

    a. Upon assignment to the unit or facility, everyone working in the unit or facility shall be oriented to the needs of people with chronic confusion or dementing illnesses. They shall have special training appropriate to their job description within 30 days of assignment to the unit or facility. (II,III)

The orientation shall be at least six hours. The following topics shall be covered:

(1) Explanation of the disease or disorder, (II,III)

(2) Symptoms and behaviors of memory-impaired people; (II,III)

(3) Progression of the disease; (II,III)

(4) Communication with CCDI residents; (II,III)

(5) Adjustment to care facility residency by the CCDI unit or facility residents and their families; (II,III)

(6) Inappropriate and problem behavior of CCDI unit or facility residents and how to deal with it; (II,III)

(7) Activities of daily living for CCDI residents (II,III)

(8) Handling combative behavior; (II,III)

(9) Stress reduction for staff and residents (II,III)

    b. Licensed nurses, certified aides, certified medication aids, social services personnel, housekeeping and activity personnel shall have a minimum of six hours of in-service training annually. This training shall be related to the needs of CCDI residents. The six-hour training shall count toward the required annual in-service training. (II,III)

ATTACHMENT D
CONTINUING EDUCATION

It is noted Attachment B is referenced Elder Affairs (321) and Attachment C is referenced Inspections and Appeals (481).

Each has specified annual continuing education requirements.

What controls are in place by the Departments of Elder Affairs or Inspections and Appeals concerning:

A. Proposed sites where the required continuing education will be scheduled and presented?
B. The subject matter to be presented? Is the subject matter to be approved before it can be presented and credit given those attending?
C. Do Elder Affairs or Inspections and Appeals require teachers or presenters of required annual continuing education subject matter to be certified or approved by their Department?

ATTACHMENT E

In the Alzheimer's Association Greater Iowa Chapter News, Spring 2010, publication it was reported there were 69,000 Iowans with Alzheimer's disease, which total was expected to rise to 77,000 by 2025. There was then disclosed, according to Facts and Figures in 2009, nearly 11 million Alzheimer caregivers in the U.S. provided 12.5 billion hours of unpaid care valued at $144 billion. It was further reported, "The uncompensated care they provide is valued at $144 billion, which is more than the Federal government spends on Medicare and Medicaid combined for people with Alzheimer's and other dementias." It was further reported, "in Iowa alone, 106,474 caregivers, provided over 121 million hours of unpaid care for a loved one with Alzheimer's or another dementia valued at more than $1.39 billion."

How concerned, interested, and informed are the people of Iowa about Alzheimer's/dementia disease?

Based upon the reported prevalence of Alzheimer's/dementia in Iowa and the predicted ascendency thereof one would conclude additional ALP/D and CCDI facilities are currently needed in Iowa, and more in the future will be needed.

In the ALP/D and CCDI facilities where Alzheimer's/dementia diseased persons are residents, who provides the care required for those residents therein? Nurses, LPNs, CMAs and CNAs, often referred to as direct care workers or caregivers provide that care.

We learn after much reading and observation an Alzheimer's diseased person's quality of life may be extended in a proper environment, staffed with persons educated and then trained to communicate, interact, using hands-on skills, learned and acquired to which skills the resident will be more receptive to, and more favorably responsive to.

According to the "2010 Alzheimer's Disease Facts and Figures," Alzheimer's disease is:

- responsible for $172 billion in annual costs in the United States
- the sixth leading cause of death in America
- currently affecting more than 5 million Americans, resulting in 11 million Alzheimer's and dementia caregivers who provide $144 billion in unpaid care for their loved ones
- a disease someone in America develops every 70 seconds and by mid-century someone will develop Alzheimer's every 33 seconds.

Questions for Physicians

Because of the personal experiences both Jo and I had commencing in 1999 and continuing through December 2006, I drafted questions which should be in the hands of all medical doctors for review before they confer with the patient and the patient's loved one concerning Alzheimer's disease.

Our experiences caused me to write a paper I entitled "Questions for Physicians," signed by me 3-20-07. I wish that someone had placed a similar Questions paper in the hands of Jo and myself back in 2001 shortly after Jo hit her ball off the 16th tee. It would have been a great help! It could be a great help to you, if you are as green, naïve, and uninformed as Jo and I initially were about dementia. Physicians should not only ask themselves these questions, but their patients should pose these questions to their physicians as well.

Questions for Physicians

My longtime patient and his spouse (in the 65-75 year age group) perceive in my patient a memory impairment; they inquire concerning the same and seek my opinion as to whether or not it could be Alzheimer's disease.

What do I their physician, know about Alzheimer's disease, or know about procedures available to determine with some accuracy whether or not my patient has Alzheimer's disease?

Taking into consideration the patient's age category what should my initial procedure be?

What inquiries of the patient and his spouse should I make initially? What history is important to establish?

How would I determine if in fact my patient has a memory impairment?

Does my patient have an attention or a language problem?

Could a prior head injury or an acute condition be the cause of the now-perceived memory impairment?

What procedures are now available that could be implemented to determine if there is in fact a memory impairment?

Would you, the family physician, proceed after obtaining the necessary history, or would you refer your patient to a neurologist, or would you first refer your patient to a neuropsychologist ?

If the neurological examination and neuropsychologist tests indicate the patient's perceived memory impairment is likely to be Alzheimer's disease, what discussion do you then have with your patient and his wife?

They want to be absolutely certain the cause of the perceived memory impairment. What further procedures are available?

Do you schedule a brain scan, an MRI, or spinal tap? What about Positron Emission Tomography (PET)?

Positron emission tomography (PET) is used in the early detection of Alzheimer's disease. Has or does anyone in Des Moines use PET to diagnose Alzheimer's disease?

In the event there is a determination your patient most likely has Alzheimer's disease, what treatment, exercise (both mental and physical), nutrition, and medication would you prescribe?

The above referred-to patient was posed to be in the 65-75 age group. For discussion, assume the patient was in the 45-55 age group; 55-65 age group, or the 75-85 age group; would your procedure be any different?

How important is early detection in the treatment of Alzheimer's disease?

What early ages is Alzheimer's disease now being detected?

Medications approved for the treatment of Alzheimer's are Aricept, Cognex, Exelon, Razadyne, and Namenda. What medication would you prescribe for your patient recently diagnosed as having Alzheimer's disease? Medications are more effective prescribed for those detected in the early stages of Alzheimer's disease.

A physician initially prescribed for his patient Aricept. For some period of time the patient had diarrhea, sometimes in public places where a toilet was not conveniently located. The patient informed the physician of the diarrhea condition and experiences. The physician suggested the patient buy Metamucil for the fiber, which the patient did. The Metamucil made no difference, the experiences continued, which the patient informed the physician of, at which time the physician informed the patient to see another physician about the diarrhea. The other physician took the patient off of Aricept to determine if that would cause the diarrhea to cease, which it did within 10-12 days; after about 20 days the other physician put the patient on Reminyl (now Razadyne) and Nemenda; no more diarrhea.

What tests are available for children of Alzheimer's diseased parents?

Those children might want to confirm at death by autopsy that their parent did in fact have Alzheimer's disease, and request that you, the parent's family physician, order an autopsy at the time of the death of their parent. Would you agree in advance of the death to then at the time of death order an autopsy? If not, why not?

If you would so agree, who would in advance, make arrangements with a neuropathologist to perform the autopsy?

Is there a neuropathologist in Des Moines? Is there one in Iowa? If so, would that specialist do the autopsy in Des Moines?

In your opinion, other than an autopsy of the brain by a neurpathologist could a valid autopsy of the brain be performed, and a valid opinion or diagnosis be reached to confirm or rule out Alzheimer's disease? If so, designate that person(s) by profession and name if you would please.

Should there be a section of practitioners who specialize in the treatment of Alzheimer's disease? "Geriatrics — Elder ailments, dementia, Alzheimer's disease." About five or so groups in Des Moines listed in the yellow pages, probably fewer than a dozen physicians.

Earlier one physician prescribed large doses of Vitamin E— Mayo Clinic and other sources suggested that practice be discontinued.

What time of day should Lexapro be given?

If it is not given at the prescribed a.m. time what effect would it have on the patient's sleep cycle?

Namenda and Razadyne, what amount of time is suggested between a.m. and p.m. doses?

What effect if, at times, there are only 7-8 hours between the a.m.-p.m. doses?

What effect if, at times, there are 15-18 hours between p.m.-a.m. meds?

Say a patient is on 10mg Lexapro and has been for over four years, that patient is in the latter stages of Alzheimer's disease, and is in excess of 80 years, do you continue the 10mg of Lexapro or do you reduce the dosage or discontinue the Lexapro?

Nameda 10mg, same question?

Razadyne 4mg, same question?

Same question re: Aricept, Cognex, and Exelon?

What do I know about care facilities such as adult day care, ALP/D, CCDI, and assisted living?

What do I know about caregivers hired to work in those facilities with Alzheimer's disease and residents; what is the capability and competence of those hired caregivers?

What is the education and training of the caregivers?

When my Alzheimer's diseased patient comes to my office for scheduled appointment accompanied by the spouse, what questions do I ask of the two; what questions do I ask of the spouse outside the presence of the patient, if any?

Am I aware of the fact that if I ask the wrong questions in the presence of my patient I could cause the patient to become excited, too stimulated, and perhaps agitated, which conditions could be harmful to patient and cause conflict with spouse?

What programs are available to persons who would consent to become personally involved in research projects?

Signed Claude Freeman, 3-20-07

Jo's Story

You will recall on January 22, 2007, when Jo was released from Methodist Hospital, Jo was taken to and became a new resident at a CCDI facility, which had opened in October 2006, Jo's chronology referenced herein commences August 8, 2008.

August 8, 2008

Jo was very tired, slouched in a chair, somewhat unresponsive. I was informed that Jo had not consumed any food that morning, nor at lunch, nor water until supper time at which time she ate well and drank some liquids. My experience caused me to conclude dehydration, UTI. Before putting Jo to bed we tried liquids, but not receptive, too tired to swallow. Around 9:45 p.m. I tried feeding her some sherbet, but she ate only a spoonful or two.

August 9, 2008

At 4:30 a.m. I went back to check on Jo, tried to get her to drink fluids, but with no success. I requested that the 11 p.m.-7 a.m. staff obtain a specimen; if they did not get one then to request the next shift, 7 a.m.-3 p.m. get the specimen. I received a call about 8:00 a.m. informing me a specimen had been taken and they were going to call someone to pick it up. I instructed the staff person on duty to keep the specimen, call Mercy and inform them that I would bring the specimen to the lab shortly, which I did. I also requested the staff person to call Mercy to inform the staff that Jo was going to be brought to the ER as soon as transportation could be arranged. That staff person was very attentive to Jo's condition and need. She wasted no time.

Jo was transported via ambulance to Mercy. I arrived shortly thereafter and had access to the ER staff. Fortunately, there was a quality staff on duty and one doctor had the foresight to order x-rays of the chest, which disclosed pneumonia in the right lung. Jo was admitted on the top floor where critical were housed. There were very noisy people in the room next door to Jo. Jo had all kinds of tubes inserted, intravenous, antibiotics, liquids, nutrition, etc. Jo kept looking at me quizzically.

August 10, 2008

August 10, 2008, we were moved to a quieter section. X-rays on that day disclosed pneumonia in both the right and left lungs. Swallowing tests were attempted to determine what caused the aspiration in the lungs—no conclusion. Every specialist in the hospital visited us and gave attention to Jo's condition. I was aware Jo had not been given any Lexapro, Razadyne, nor Namenda during her stay. A day or so before she was released I suggested to her regular staff doctors that we discontinue the use of the Alzheimer's medications. They agreed to discontinue Razadyne and Namenda, but felt that Lexapro, an anti-depressant, be continued.

August 19, 2008

Jo was returned to her CCDI care facility around 2:00 p.m. this date, after ten or so tough days of uncertainty. The director of the CCDI unit was at the hospital to visit with Jo and her doctors and received copies of instructions and directions to follow on Jo's release. The director said to Jo several times, "Jo, I will see you when you get back." Jo then responded in a clear, but soft and polite voice, "I'm sure you will."

It was not determined during Jo's stay in the hospital what caused the lungs aspiration. They did several swallow tests, but none were conclusive. Jo was placed on a puree diet, later changed to a soft diet, as there was some concern that involuntary muscles were not functioning as they should in the chewing and swallowing process, but once the food reached the area of the esophagus and involuntary muscles took over, the digestive process appeared to be quite normal.

January 25, 2009

(Sunday) The nurse informed me the director had suggested to her that she discuss with me the inclination to cease giving Jo the thickened juices and instead give Jo a juice pill, which would be better for Jo. I inquired how or why the juice pill would be better. The nurse then explained that Jo was given the thickened juices because of a difficulty in swallowing, which condition I was well aware of. When Jo was hospitalized in August 2008, they did swallow tests, which disclosed that when the chewing process was stimulated and the food went into the esophagus and started out of the esophagus, the digestive process was normal as usual. The involuntary muscle process took over to complete the digestive and then the elimination process.

By sipping, and then by experiencing the familiar taste of the thickened orange juice, does that process assist in maintaining a continued muscle memory, especially to stimulate Jo in chewing and swallowing foods that go into the esophagus and out into the digestive system?

More questions immediately came to mind.

I informed the nurse I would think about the suggested procedure, mull it over, and get back to her on Monday. At which time she informed me she would be off on Monday, but back on Tuesday, at which time we could talk or visit again.

Why now, after four or five months, discontinue the thickened juices and substitute a juice pill?

What are the reasons for the proposed change?

Is it too onerous for the staff to spoon feed Jo the juice, or have her sip the thickened juice?

Is there too much spillage when the staff endeavors to get Jo to sip or drink the juice?

Which is more advantageous for Jo, the thickened juice or the juice pill?

Which of the two will better hydrate Jo? —Hydration is an important factor.

Where does digestion of the thickened juice commence, then at what sections of the body is it absorbed before the remains are expelled or urinated from the body?

Same questions apply to the juice pill.

Which, then, would be more advantageous to the health of Jo?

One can read on the thickened juice container, the ingredients of the thickened juice. What are the ingredients therein?

What are the ingredients in the juice pill?

Compare.

Which is the most nutritious?

After the juice pill is swallowed and the outer cover is being dissolved, what is the content being released into the body at what stages and locations?

(I was then informed that if the juice pill was given, it would have been crushed and given with applesauce.)

How much water or liquid would a person consuming a juice pill have to drink to cause the contents of the juice pill to be as effective in the body as the thickened juice?

Does the juice pill have a flavor or taste similar to thickened juice, which actually stimulates the person being fed to consume more juice, food, etc.?

From what source does one acquire the proposed juice pill? Thickened juice? (I was informed the juice pill was purchased over-the-counter, non-prescribed.)

Thickened juice is apparently a food item, part of Jo's diet menu.

Is the juice pill a non-prescription cost? (I was advised the cost of the same goes on our monthly billing.)

I can easily make decisions when I am fully informed. I'm not making busy work and I haven't formed an opinion on thickened juice or juice pills. I only desire to make a prudent decision.

Addendum:

Jo has a tendency to want to chew a pill rather than swallow it. Crushing the pill may affect its intended purpose or use.

January 28, 2009

Back in October 2008, juice was watered one-half and one-half to lessen sugar intake.

New diet: One-half portions, no sweets, no desserts, fruit instead—blueberries and cranberries special ingredients that fight possible UTI germs, eliminates UTI germs in urinary tract. Jo only gets cranberry juice—go back to regular cranberry juice, not watered down, thickened cranberry juice, no juice pill.

March 2, 2009

Friday night Jo had a large stool and could not eliminate all the bowel; two CNAs came into the bathroom to assist in getting Jo into bed at which time they became informed of removing a dangling stool. They went to get the CMA who declined to endeavor to remove the dangling stool and left Jo on the stool for a long period. Jo could not get the stool to move, took her bath, still no stool removal, at which time the CMA suggested a suppository could be inserted, which was at 8:45-9:00 p.m.

I remained there until 11:15 p.m., no movement, at which time I discovered that Jo had wet the bed. The CNAs came, changed the pads. The next morning Jo had a small bowel movement.

Three or so years prior to 1957 when I first met Jo, she was returning to Des Moines from her family farm in Adams County. In the vicinity of Patterson, Iowa, an elderly gentleman suddenly pulled out from a country road onto the highway in front of Jo. She swerved her vehicle in an attempt to avoid striking the other vehicle, resulting in Jo's vehicle going off the highway and into a ditch where the front of her vehicle collided with a culvert or some object in the ditch. Jo's chin struck the steering wheel with great force, resulting in a severe laceration of the chin and caused considerable damage to her teeth. It was necessary to replace three or four damaged teeth located in the left upper side of Jo's face immediately in front of the rear molars with a partial.

March 12, 2009

The director of the CCDI facility telephoned me at 4:30 p.m. or 4:45 p.m. to inform me that Jo's partial denture was missing and that she, staff, and the maintenance people had been searching everywhere for it. She wanted me to know before my visit after supper. (It was later reported that they were not aware that the denture was not in place until getting Jo seated for lunch.) All kinds of questions popped into my mind, such as: Who dressed Jo? Who removed the denture from the pink box? Who did what with the denture thereafter? Who fed Jo breakfast? After breakfast, who removed the bib, wiped Jo's face, checked for food deposits in her mouth, hydrated Jo, after breakfast toilet procedure, activity period, to bed, nap procedure? Between breakfast and lunch were clothes changed? Were laundry and cleaning people alerted—put on notice? Who prepared Jo for lunch and actually seated Jo? Who fed Jo at lunch—hydrated Jo?

Must establish routine for early a.m. placement of denture in Jo's mouth. The nurse or CMA on 7 a.m.-3 p.m.: What was her routine for placing denture in Jo's mouth? Why wasn't that procedure followed? Or was it followed?

Question: Who, and when, and what time actually determined Jo's denture was not in place? What procedure was implemented at time of discovery? Now, one day later, and after reflection by all, what additional search can be made to endeavor to locate Jo's denture? Is it in the laundry? Someone's medical box or other personal container in nurses' station? Beauty shop? Other resident's room? Do not quit looking for denture!

I have now been told CNA waking and dressing Jo each morning would remove the partial denture from the pink container where I place it every night, rinse it, and put a paper towel around it or over it, then wheel Jo to the nurses' station where CNA hand or give nurse there the denture, which nurse will place a salve, prescribed to treat a small yeast infection in the roof of Jo's mouth, on the top of the denture; then insert the denture in Jo's mouth. Apparently the nurse was not at her station so the CNA left the denture on the desk of the nurse, then placed Jo at her table for breakfast. The nurse received a telephone call which required her to leave immediately for family or personal reason. It is inconceivable that someone could pick up a weighted paper towel or Kleenex from a desktop in the nurse's station and toss it into a wastebasket or whatever action occurred.

Now I am confronted with what will happen if the partial denture is not found. Jo is sensitive about her teeth, especially the partial denture. I was informed at the outset by the director of the CCDI unit that the care facility would pay costs of replacing the denture.

I called our dentist to inform him of the lost denture. He instructed me he would not see Jo that day, I was to call later to confirm that the denture could not be found then a representative in his office would set the first appointment two weeks subsequent to the date I was calling, to allow a spot in the roof of the mouth to heal. Impression would probably be made at that first appointment. There would be four appointments, the first and last at his office, possibly the second and third at the CCDI facility. The procedure would take about four and a half weeks.

The director of the CCDI facility was to check Jo's mouth to determine if it was healed.

We must not cause Jo to become alarmed—she is very sensitive about her partial denture. If she becomes aware that the denture is lost or not in her mouth, she will become very closed-mouthed, won't eat, talk, etc. Make sure she gets through the first two-week waiting period at least.

March 13, 2009

On Friday, March 13, 2009, at 9:00 a.m., I visited with the CCDI director and activity director. I had a good visit—they read my series of questions, observations, suggestions, and I gave them copies. We visited, and made other suggestions.

They then disclosed to me in detail the effort exerted to locate the denture, including the fact that the director and maintenance manager tromped through the dumpsters and emptied bags looking for the denture. They were going to search further today (the 13th).

Later I called the dentist—office closed—I left word that the denture had not been found. About 2:50 p.m. the dentist called and suggested next week he was pretty busy and would be out of town next Thursday; then said he might get us in on Wednesday. I then informed him that he had told me yesterday that he didn't want to see Jo for two weeks—that he wanted to let the roof of her mouth heal before seeing Jo and commencing the impression. Then he began telling me he had said something different, not even mentioning the spot in the roof of Jo's mouth. I then told him exactly what he had said yesterday. Then he said he had time to see Jo on the 23rd of March at 11:00 a.m., a one-hour appointment. He would clean her teeth and probably do an impression, then other appointments would be made.

For some reason, he then wanted to know what transportation service we would use to transport Jo to his office. I informed him the director would make those arrangements depending on who was available. I then telephoned the director to inform her of the conversation with the dentist and of the appointment scheduled. The director will now proceed to make arrangements and will go with us to the dentist's office on the 23rd.

March 18, 2009

I met with the director of the CCDI facility and the activities director and gave them a copy of the following:

1. Presently it would appear that Jo is not aware that her denture is not in place.

2. The appointment to clean her teeth, inspect the infected area, and do an impression and during the hour-long appointment conversation between the hygienist, doctor, and staff, Jo could very well become aware, then or later in the day after the appointment, that her denture is not in her mouth.

3. If she did have the awareness she would be very disturbed.

4. Subsequent to the initial appointment, there would be three later appointments, two proposed to be at the CCDI facility, the last at the dentist's office.

5. It was suggested initially that it would be a four-and-a-half week process.

6. Fitting the denture is very important; conditions not visibly apparent to the dentist could not be communicated or conveyed by Jo to the dentist with accuracy. It could become a great annoyance, and/or a great distraction for Jo.

Neither staff nor I want Jo to be in pain, annoyed, or distracted by any substance, object, or condition.

7. Presently, Jo is, at times, quite animated, much like herself, eats her puree diet quite well; she laughs and smiles and speaks as if she was confident that her denture was in place. We will do nothing presently to cause her to become aware it is not in place.

8. Cancel the scheduled appointment.

9. Claude will meet with the director and the director of activities on 3/19/09, to confer, convey his thoughts, get their thoughts and reactions.

10. If soon Jo is made aware that her denture is not in place, and she has an adverse reaction, which conversation and explanation regarding the absence of the denture does not relieve her of the adverse reaction, then we will probably proceed to have a new denture made, taking into account all the conditions at that place in time.

11. Hopefully, the CCDI facility does not demand the procedure be done presently.

12. Claude will call the dentist office after meeting with the director and the activity director to cancel the 3-23-09 scheduled appointment.

13. In the event the dentist would call the CCDI facility to confer with anyone concerning the cancelation or Jo's status or condition, etc., no authority is given for such communication presently.

14. Beauty shop: Jo may need a hair cut soon. The hairdresser should be cautioned not to mention partial denture

absence or cause Jo to look at herself in the mirror.

15. The director and/or Jo's attending physician should tactfully examine or inspect (look at) the roof of Jo's mouth to make certain it is healed or is healing.

16. Wouldn't it be great if the denture was, at this late date, recovered?

17. Claude, between 2:45 and 2:50 p.m. on Thursday 3-19-09 called the dentist's office, got answering service, a voice answered, leaving a message, in substance, "We are out of town, the office is closed Thursday, we will be back in the office on Monday the 23rd." I then left the following message, "Currently, Jo has shown no awareness that her partial denture is not in place. After observing her for a week now without her partial denture in place, and after much thought, it is most prudent I cancel the appointment scheduled Monday the 23rd at 11:00 a.m.—if time and conditions cause a change in my thinking we will then confer with the dentist. Calling today will allow you some time to schedule someone else for Monday at 11:00 a.m."

18. Does anyone on the CCDI staff know about the appointment for Monday? If so, there should be no discussion with staff regarding the appointment or the cancellation.

As of October 8, 2010, Jo has not exhibited an awareness the partial denture is not in place. Jo continues to eat, or be fed, a soft diet and thickened liquids that were prescribed subsequent to her hospitalization commencing August 9, 2008, where it was determined Jo should be fed a puree diet, later a soft food diet.

April 20, 2009

Letter from staff or resident physician that she would be starting a Preventative Medicine Fellowship at Mayo Clinic in July, which would be a two-year program with many exciting new things to learn that had promise to improve patient care for the future. Among other opportunities, that person would be involved with the Mayo Clinic Health Policy Center that works with Washington D.C. to improve national health care. It was that person's goal to focus on adult and geriatric preventative medicine to bring to the forefront how we can keep people healthy instead of just fixing health problems as they arise.

April 28, 2009

Confer with the director of the CCDI facility regarding CNA assistance in toileting Jo, etc.

April 30, 2009

Subsequent to discontinuing Razadyne and Namenda, shortly before 8-19-08 when Jo was a patient at Mercy Hospital, it was my observation that Jo had more energy and her cognitive ability was more acute. I raised the question, "Does Jo really require an expert in Alzheimer's disease?"

May 21, 2009

The following are excerpts from correspondence I directed to the departing physician who would be starting a fellowship at Mayo clinic in July.

There is not much time left between now, May 21, and the first of July. I do not know when your successor will assume patient care at the CCDI facility. Now, soon and immediately I must make prudent decisions concerning Jo's future medical care and treatment. I am of the opinion a personal discussion with you would enable me to make prudent decisions concerning Jo's future medical care and treatment. Therefore, I would appreciate an opportunity to meet with you as soon as possible.

Since August, 2008, when certain medications were discontinued, Jo has, over time, shown greater awareness, and her visual, physical, and verbal responses are more spontaneous, natural, and appropriate. Jo is currently doing certain exercises with staff on certain mornings. Staff have reported walking with Jo in the hall at times to some extent. Recently, as we were sitting and visiting, or when I was pushing Jo in her chair, she has endeavored and has attempted to and has crossed one leg over the other, which really surprised me. She is very quick to reach out to touch or grab on to things that have come to her attention as she is being pushed for a ride in her chair. All are positive, animated, visually perceived, natural, physically coordinated responses. Presently, I question whether Jo requires a specialist or an expert in care and treatment of Alzheimer's disease. Medications currently prescribed seem to be very effective. I would not anticipate nor expect a need for a change in those medications, nor for a change in the dosage thereof. I need your counsel soon. Thank you for your consideration.

Sincerely yours, Claude Freeman.

Subsequently, a physician from the departing physician's office assumed the care of Jo.

July 5, 2009

Jo's birthday! Jo, assisted by two CNAs, walked from bathroom and activity area to a wooden bench in Boulevard Place where our son Hugh was waiting.

The CCDI facility schedules care conferences. Persons attending usually are a person from social services, the nutritionist and the director of the CCDI facility meeting with a family member of the Alzheimer's diseased resident, during which meeting the care plan of the resident will be reviewed and revised with the members of the interdisciplinary care team mentioned above. Each conference usually lasts 20 minutes, or longer, if necessary. A letter is directed to the family member of the resident who generally attended the scheduled care conference. Notification of the scheduled care conference is mailed to the representative along with a Care Plan Conference Questionnaire. I filled out the questionnaire and mailed it timely to the representative from social services prior to the conference scheduled Monday, July 13, 2009. The questionnaire lists areas of concern such as dietary concerns, social services concerns, personal care, staff accommodations, environment, programming/activities, other. For that July 13 scheduled care conference, I responded as follows:

Dietary concerns: Weight—liquid—puree diet—calorie count—liquid Colace—bowel and bowel movement—exercise—walk—leg exercise

Personal care: Arms rigidity—hand closing—dressing and undressing—bruises—socks and bras wrong-side out

Staff accommodations: Bib—juice stains on shirt

Environment: Constant monitoring of thermostats

Programming/activities: The haircut—hermit crab—red fish—Jo very aware, perceptive communication

For that scheduled care conference, I submitted to those present at the care conference the following typed:

1. Why is weight so high–155 pounds? Feeding liquid, puree type diet, caloric control. CNA has been faithful to exercise and walk Jo, and now includes a leg exercise which will assist bowel movement.

2. Should the liquid Colace be given every day? Given basically a soft or liquid diet at every meal, given a liquid stool softener daily, will the bowel become a so-called regular bowel movement? The bowel is rather large in volume presently, heavy in content, by appearance, and its consistency could be compared, possibly, to peanut butter, and it does not seem to fall apart in the stool, or fall off objects it adheres to. Presently, bowel movements are a bit more regular, it seems. Maybe CNA exercises are a factor.

3. At times Jo's left hand is quite tightly closed, even when sitting, lying in bed. It is not a conscious effort I am certain. I wash her hands after dinner each evening. After I wash her right hand, I take her left hand and it is rigid, tightly clasped. I tell her I will wash her hand, but we must open our hand and extend our fingers. I put the warm cloth on top of her hand to wipe there and as I put her hand in mine, she opens her hand fully to be wiped. Undressing her later, when I am removing her top, we remove her right arm from her top first, telling her we are removing her arm from the sleeve, and how easy that process was. Then we go to the left, finding the hand and arm somewhat rigid, I remind her how easy it will be to remove this arm if we just relax and then open our hand so the sleeve will slide off. I would assume that similar hand and arm rigidity occur during dressing. It takes patience, but it is not an intentional act of resistance by Jo in the dressing or undressing process. When I brush her teeth in the evening as she is lying in bed she is very cooperative once I tell her what a good job she is doing, keeping her mouth open wide, etc.

4. There are bruises on both of Jo's arms and legs, no indication that Jo is bruising herself—if so when is she striking

what? The wheelchair seems well padded. Socks are on Jo's arms and legs.

5. Bra! Minor issue—just curious how one female person could or would put a bra on another female person that is obviously wrong-side out, more times than once!

6. I see large bibs on residents being fed, which cover the area just below the chin and down the chest to the waist. Frequently Jo gets juice stains on her tops in the area below the chin, even though she is being fed generally by spoon.

7. Haircut.

8. Hermit crab, little red fish in the aquarium in the atrium.

9. Jo very aware, perceptive.

October 11, 2009

Care Plan Conference Questionnaire remarks dated 10-11-09 are:

(At 5:00 a.m. on 10-14-09, being spelled correctly and supplemented.)

Dietary concerns: What is Jo's current weight? Jo is basically on a puree or soft diet. What portions of food are given to Jo at each of her three meals? When I get Jo ready for bed each night I note the increase of fat from her armpits to her crotch. That section of her body has become unbelievably obese. Her breasts are twice their normal size. We have gone from small to medium and recently to large shirts or tops. Bras from 38 to 38-40 and recently a 40-42 size bra. Pants from a size 12 petite to a 14, and now, for some time, to a 16 petite.

Liquid Colace is given each night around 7:15 p.m. The odor or taste of the liquid Colace is softened or made more palatable mixed with applesauce, then followed by 6 to 8 teaspoons of thickened cranberry or orange juice. Colace (liquid) must be mixed and given in the described way, otherwise it tastes awful and unless mixed properly huge bubbles pop out of Jo's mouth and a bad, physically exerting cough will commence.

Thickened juice, given several times daily. What calories or fattening agents are consumed?

Colace is effective. Jo has large bowel movements with some regularity. Do meal portions have an effect on Jo processing food swallowed, half-chewed, and the ultimate bowel elimination thereof?

The CNA has been very attentive of Jo, working on Jo's strengths and walking Jo for exercise, and in an effort to help Jo ambulate better and more often. If I can assist the CNA in her efforts to exercise Jo and to ambulate Jo, tell me, inform me when to be there.

Obesity is not good! What can be done to lessen it and not allow the propensity to continue?

Supplement: Monday night, 10-12-09, on my arrival at 6:20 p.m. or so, I was greeted by a CNA who informed me, in substance, that Jo really ate well. She had fruit, mangoes, whole food and chewed it right down. I then took Jo down to her room, got her ready for our usual trip downstairs, then back upstairs where each evening around 7:10 p.m. Colace is given. The CMA on duty mixed the Colace with a snow-cone-looking substance. On this particular evening the CMA, using a teaspoon, filled the spoon excessively full, probably three times the amount the liquid applesauce would need and fed the contents of the cup into Jo's mouth at a rather rapid pace. During the process a bubble popped out of Jo's mouth. As soon as the Colace was given, thickened juice was given at the same pace. I always wheel Jo around for a few minutes, or sit and talk with her a bit after the Colace has been given to allow the Colace to be processed in the digestive system. I then took Jo down to her room to get her ready to be placed on the stool and get her ready for her Monday night bath. I barely got the foot pads off her wheelchair when she began to cough. I patted her on her back and tried to get her to breathe. The cough stopped briefly and then greater effort was being made to cough or clear her airways. I wheeled her up the hall to where the CMA was sitting with other residents. I then took Jo into the dining area where coughing continued. The CMA came to that area at which time Jo was exerting great effort to clear her airways. Her face, neck, and head were very red as her muscles therein were responding to her involuntary response to the conditions the Colace created. A couple spoons of heated thickened water was given to clear Jo's airways. The coughing abated. It was suggested that Jo remain in the dining area for 15 more minutes, which we did. I then took Jo to her room at which time I kneeled down to remove the metal footrest from Jo's chair. Jo coughed once, then a second time very strongly, at which time moisture from the cough hit the top of my head. I could observe the fatigue that was setting in, and informed the CMA that it was my suggestion that I get Jo ready for bed and that we forego the scheduled bath and suggested the next-day crew could give Jo a bath, to which the CMA agreed. I put Jo to bed and remained there until 9:15 p.m. or so.

I arrived last night, 10-13-09, regular time. Jo was quite animated. We did our usual trip and then came back for the Colace and applesauce at 7:15 p.m. The regular CMA was on duty. That CMA gave her regular mixture of applesauce and Colace in a teaspoon at a sensible pace, followed by thickened cranberry juice, without incidence.

I inquired if Jo had been given a bath during the 7 a.m.-3 p.m. shift and was informed there was no record of it, I suggested Jo be given a bath, as she had her last bath Friday, 10-09-09. It was agreed, so Jo had her bath and had fallen asleep by 8:20 p.m.

I thanked the staff for a good night as I departed about 8:30 p.m., knowing Jo was then resting well.

I was extremely concerned when Jo was coughing so laboriously 10-12-09, that she would burst a blood vessel or artery, or cause serious damage elsewhere, and it may have. I mention this now as we must get a prescribed process for mixing the Colace with a substance that will make it more palatable, and a prescribed procedure for spooning the mixture in a manner that will not cause a similar incident from 10-12-09 to reoccur. All CMAs should follow that prescribed process. The reason we are using the liquid Colace is that Jo too frequently would not or could not swallow the pill—she would then bite the pill, crushing it before swallowing it. Perhaps we could inquire if it would be possible, without affecting the integrity of the pill, to crush the pill then place the crushed pill in applesauce, and give it to Jo. That

151

process would probably eliminate all the problems associated with giving the liquid Colace.

Thank you all for allowing a concerned, attentive, and dedicated spouse to answer the Care Plan Questionnaire in this manner. My intentions are constructive not obstructive.

Signed Claude Freeman, 10-14-09

My notes at the conclusion of that meeting were as follows:
A. Good meeting.
B. Inquire what the particular CMA uses for a mix-Colace.
C. Formula by everyone.
D. Physical therapy—set of exercises Claude Freeman can assist with ambulation and exercises the physical therapist prescribes as approved by the treating physician.
E. Suggest reducing the dosage of Lasix if no suppository is used in the previous month.

October 22, 2009

COLACE:

Sometime ago, for conditions then existing, Colace (docusate sodium) a stool softener was prescribed in capsule (pill) form. A pill would be placed in a teaspoon of applesauce and then spooned into Jo's mouth. There would be times Jo swallowed the mixture immediately, then there were times Jo sensed a lump (pill) at which time Jo would begin to chew the lump in the applesauce, biting into the pill and crushing it. Frequent experiences such as this caused a change from a capsule to prescribed liquid Colace. Side effects associated with liquid Colace are a bitter taste, throat irritation, and nausea. Rash has occurred. Jo has always liked good applesauce, for that reason applesauce was to be mixed nightly with the prescribed liquid Colace to make it more palatable. When mixed properly, little or no reaction when the mixture was spooned into her mouth or when swallowing or after swallowing.

Monday, October 12, 2009, and Sunday, October 18, 2009, a staff person elected to use Lyon's Ready Care Instant Food Thickener, which is basically a modified cornstarch, rather than, or in place of, applesauce. Previously on October 14, I referenced the October 12 incident in Care Plan Conference, corrected and supplemented questionnaire remarks. The Sunday, October 18, experience was similar, if not worse. The coughing episode began after only a partial dose was given.

If the applesauce was used to lessen the bad taste of the liquid Colace, making it more palatable, and easier for Jo to swallow in its liquid form, in which form the prescribed dosage would go down her throat and into the esophagus then to where involuntary muscles move the dosage more quickly downward through the digestive tract. This process would less likely result in any throat irritation.

Cornstarch is a binder used as a thickening agent in cooking; a binder for puddings, or similar foods, or as a thickener for sauces, stews, etc. The thickener is viscous; viscosity is defined as the state or quality of being viscous. In physics the internal fluid resistance of a substance caused by molecular attraction, which makes it resist a tendency to flow. It is presumed the staff person poured the prescribed dosage of Colace into the selected cup where the thickener was added and then spoon-mixed the two substances to bind. The Colace would then no longer be in its prescribed liquid form. The elected mixture would not eliminate the bitter taste, nor make the dosage more palatable, nor would it protect against possible irritation. The prescribed liquid

Colace, after the thickener was mixed with it, became less fluid; it was then no longer readily flowing.

In that communication I thanked the director of the CCDI facility for allowing me to visit the afternoon after the 10-18-09 experience and referenced experiences, and I thanked the director for the current endeavor to arrive at a proper mixture of applesauce with the prescribed dosage of liquid Colace. The proper mixture should eliminate the stressful, coughing episodes.

Around 10-25-09 I observed a cup sitting on Jo's lavatory in which was a mouth-washing substance, which piqued my curiosity! Could Jo now gargle and spit out the contents? Could she sip juice after the Colace-applesauce was spoon given? Simple questions.

Subsequently, I observed at a noon meal, two different staff persons having Jo drink juice from a glass tilted by that staff person. After the evening meal on the same day, I observed Jo's juice glass was empty. I inquired of the staff person if Jo drank all her juice; I was informed, yes, she drank it all. I inquired if she drank it from the glass; she said yes, she did a good job. I was informed that is permissible, but not sipping through a straw.

Three months ago, 7-14-09, I noted in a paper I wrote Jo's weight was 155 pounds; now three months later, 10-09, she has gained 11 pounds to 166 pounds, some 40 pounds above her usual weight of 122-126 pounds.

Meals? Meal portions for each of the three meals, Saturday, 10-31-09, saucer-sized (turned upside down) portion of tuna melt, cauliflower, assume cottage cheese; staff kept spooning in what was on plate when half of the portions served would have been more than sufficient. Were the tuna, cauliflower, and cottage cheese thickened too? Jo always controlled her food intake. She naturally never stuffed nor overate. Unfortunately, she is not aware, presently, of the amount of food being placed in her mouth three times a day.

If all her three meals each day are similar portions as served 10-31-09, plus thickened juice or water, are fed to Jo each day, that is the cause of her weight increase. **We have to limit Jo's food intake!** Otherwise, she will not lose weight, weight gain will continue. Too much food may be a cause of large, difficult bowel movements, requiring Colace.

I met with the CCDI director and the activity director on Monday 11-02-09 regarding weight and feeding portions.

November 6, 2009

This paper is typed 11-05-09 from notes used during 11-02-09 meeting with the CCDI director and activity director:

Diet and Weight

Diet and weight have been topics at Care Plan Conferences.

My wife has gained 31 pounds since she has been a resident in CCDI facility.

Toward the end of October, 2009, her weight was recorded at 166 pounds. A paper I provided 10-11-09 entitled Care Plan Conference Questionnaire Remarks, I related, among other things, "We have gone from small to medium and recently to large tops; bras from 38-40 recently to a 40-42 bra; pants from a 12 petite to a 14, and now, for some time a 16 petite." It is apparent my wife, Jo Freeman, is being overfed daily. I am advised, in substance, a statute or regulation mandates a specific meal or daily caloric quantity for care facilities residents, including the residents in this CCDI facility. What is the source of, and the citation of the statute or regulation? Are there exceptions written in the statute or regulation? If so, under what conditions or circumstances can the care facility nutritionist prescribe less calories to a particular resident than mandated by statute or regulations?

In other words, does the regulation apply to everyone in the facility, or exceptions? Some residents in the facility may be 50 years of age, ambulatory, active, and can participate in all activities, have no chewing or swallowing difficulties, are not required to take a daily laxative, are not required to drink thickened juice and water, etc. Would the 80–90-year-old sedentary non-ambulatory residents who have other infirmities be required to consume the same food portions as the 50-year-old referenced above?

What if records now disclose that by rigidly complying with the caloric statute or regulation the 80–90-year-old sedentary residents in the facility gained nine-and-a-half pounds in the first 12 months of residency in the facility, then gained an additional six-and-a-half pounds in the next five months of residency; a total of 16 pounds in the first 17 months of residency in the facility? What if records disclosed that from March 2007, to the last week in October 2009, a total of 31 months, the weight of the 80–90-year-old residents went from 135 pounds to 166 pounds, a total of 31 pounds gained; would you persist in feeding those residents the same amount of food daily to comply with a statute or regulation? What if those residents live another five years, that's 60 months more, feeding them as you did the previous 31 months, those residents would then weigh 220 pounds!

It is obvious too much food is being fed continuously to a person, who at 166 pounds is 40 pounds heavier than her normal weight of 122-126 pounds. We must now determine how the 166-pound person can lose weight, not continue to gain a pound each month!

Signed by Claude Freeman, 11-06-09

I inquired as of this date (11-05-09), "have the three daily meal portions being served and fed to Jo been reduced subsequent to November 2, 2009?" The director responded, no, already receiving reduced portions. "Since Jo is not ambulatory, is basically sedentary, have all staff persons been informed that Jo is not required or compelled to eat entirely all the portions of the food placed before her?" Answered, yes, discussed with nurses and CNAs.

November 9, 2009

Meeting with dietitian, director of CCDI and activity director.

At 2:30 a.m. this date, November 10, 2009, I woke up reflecting on things communicated during our meeting yesterday. I have tried to rationalize why a solution was not amicably reached. It is now 5:00 a.m. as I write this to each of you.

For the July Care Plan Conference I circulated the following:

Why is weight so high—155 pounds? Feeding liquid, puree-type diet, caloric control. CNA has been faithful to exercise and walk Jo, and now includes a leg exercise, which will assist bowel movement.

Should the liquid Colace be given every day? Given basically a soft or liquid diet at every meal, given a liquid stool softener daily, will the bowel become a so-called regular bowel movement? The bowel is rather large in volume presently, heavy in content, by appearance, and its consistency could be compared, possibly, to peanut butter, and it does not seem to fall apart in the stool, or fall off objects it adheres to. Presently, bowel movements are a bit more regular, it seems. Maybe CNA exercises are a factor.

Let us concentrate on Jo's weight from July, 2009, to October, 2009, during which period of time Jo's weight increased from 155 pounds to 166 pounds!

From July 2009, through October 2009, and continuing into November 2009, the CNA has continued to work with Jo, exercising and ambulating, which I greatly appreciate. Jo had not been totally sedentary (fixed to one spot as a barnacle) during the three month's time from July to October. If the CNA had not been exercising and ambulating Jo during that July-October three-month period of time, would Jo's weight increase more than 11 pounds?

Jo's Story: Who Is Caring?

Why did Jo's weight increase 11 pounds from July to October?

Food fed to Jo during that three-month period caused Jo to gain 11 pounds from 155 pounds to 166 pounds!

I regret our meeting yesterday was not pleasant or productive. I had such high hopes answers and proposed plans would be conveyed that would cause me to walk out of that meeting knowing the dietitian had a solution to the prior three-month food portions and food consumption that caused the 11-pound gain. I therefore was terribly disappointed and frustrated.

Plan directed to the dietician:

Now that you have been made aware of the weight Jo gained during the three-month period of time between July and October, as a dietitian, for a diet kitchen (a kitchen as in a hospital where special diets for patients are planned by a dietitian) please inform the CCDI director and the activity director and me, in writing, your plan and recommendations.

Signed by Claude Freeman 11-10-09

To dietitian, CCDI director and activity director:

At our 11-09-09 meeting I requested from the dietitian and the CCDI director, written copies of requested materials, information, plans and/or instructions. The requests were made to each of you separately at different times during the meeting and when I made the requests, each of you immediately made notes on the specific request directed to you.

Orally, subsequently, after our meeting, I was informed concentrated meal planning had commenced and instructions re: portions to be served and actual food to be fed or consumed by Jo implemented.

Subsequent to 11-09-09, I would presume the dietitian gave written instructions to the person(s) in charge in the kitchen re: daily meals planned for Jo's breakfast, lunch, and dinner, including any caloric references, specific nutrients, foods not to be given or included, etc.

Secondly, I would presume the dietitian gave written instructions to the kitchen staff re: foods, liquids, and portions thereof to be placed on Jo's plate to be set before her in the CCDI facility at breakfast, lunch, and dinner.

Thirdly, I would presume the dietitian provided to the director of the CCDI facility a copy of those written instructions referenced immediately above, which written instructions would enable the director and all staff persons in the CCDI facility to become precisely informed concerning the dietitian's prescribed, nutritional foods, and portions thereof to be served to Jo at three daily mealtimes.

(Directed to the director of the CCDI facility) I would be sure the director has given the CCDI facility staff written instructions concerning Jo's diet, weight gain, food portions previously fed to Jo, foods now being prescribed, portions being placed on Jo's plate in the kitchen, then placed before her at mealtime, food amounts to be fed to Jo at each mealtime setting, pace of feeding Jo her food and the consumption of liquids.

Everyone involved in the care and feeding of Jo must be informed accurately and informatively by the dietitian, in writing, concerning nutritional foods and portions thereof, to be served and fed to Jo. Receiving and circulating the requested written materials in the manner suggested is the single, most effective process; all concerned, including me, Jo's husband, and Jo's treating physician will be informed accurately and informatively. Every responsible, interested and concerned individual will then be on the same page! Please provide, in writing, requests made.

Signed Claude H. Freeman, 11-19-09, 12:30 p.m.

November 19, 2009

The dietitian issued the following:

Re: Josephine Freeman

The following measures were put into place:
Breakfast meal would include

½ cup hot cereal,

One container yogurt,

Nectar thickened liquids

Lunch and supper meals would include

#20 level scoop of meat

#20 level scoop of vegetables

#20 level scoop of fruit

Nectar thickened liquids

No potatoes, rice or noodles are to be given. No casseroles, bread or rolls or any other starch-type items are to be offered at any meals.

In discussion with the director of the CCDI facility, a blood specimen will be drawn one month subsequent to these meal changes to determine if these restrictions are impacting her nutritional status. Skin will continue to be closely monitored to make sure she is having no skin breakdown due to meal changes.

Oral mucosa will continue to be monitored to assure she is adequately hydrated and that her gums and tongue remain pink and moist. MD has been notified of the changes that have been made.

Upon review of the weight book it is noted that she lost 1# last week and 1# this week. Her weight will continue to be monitored weekly by this writer. If the weight drops more than 3# in one week, changes will again be made to make sure the weight does not come off too quickly.

I will not allow Jo's nutritional status to be compromised and I will follow closely.

Signed by the dietitian.

Received by Claude Freeman the evening of 11-19-09.

I received the following from the director of the CCDI:

Attention all CNAs and Nurses:

Jo Freeman has been experiencing weight gains and related to this we must change the way we go about assisting her.

Her husband, Claude, has made the request that we try to avoid over-feeding Jo.

After she has consumed a minimum of over 50% of the portions served, please assess how she is eating, assess if she has slowed with her chewing and how quickly she opens her mouth for additional bites.

If you note any of the above noted behaviors, or if she appears full, it is appropriate to assist her in consuming all her fluids and then stop.

Please call or stop by with any concern.

Signed by the Director of the CCDI facility.

Received by Claude Freeman 11-19-2009.

January 6, 2010

Jo's treating physician came to the CCDI care facility to see and examine Jo. After examining her, he ordered, among other things, she be given 2,000 cc of liquid per day and ordered a chest x-ray.

January 6, 2010

The treating physician telephoned me to inform me he received and read the radiologist's report, which disclosed an enlarged area suggestive of congestive heart failure, fluid in the lower-right area. The treating physician prescribed a water pill (Lasix) commencing 1-08-10, one pill each day for three days, expecting or intending for Jo to lose five pounds of fluid each day. Weigh Jo at the time first pill is given, then weigh her each of the following two days to monitor the effect of the pills.

January 8, 2010

On this day Jo weighed 160 pounds. (Of note, 1-08-10, morning before first Lasix was given, Jo had a large bowel movement.)

January 9, 2010

It was reported to me this morning, Jo wet twice during the night of 1-08-10, then when awakened early morning 1-09-10, before breakfast, her bed was wet, two tinkles after breakfast, then around 11:15 a.m., bed wet again. Good lunch, then about 1:00 p.m. wet her pants; 9:15 p.m., wet bed. Staff informed me that was the eighth time she urinated on 1-09. Weight at noon on 1-09 was, I believe, 160 or 161 pounds.

January 10, 2010

At 9:30 a.m., asleep. Reported she ate good breakfast; weight 163 pounds. When I left at 9:30 p.m. on 1-10, it was reported between a.m. and by 4:00 p.m. Jo had four tinkles and by 9:30 p.m., for the day she had eight tinkles and weighed 163 pounds.

It is presumed more than 27 separate urination experiences occurred from the time the first Lasix was given and until being awakened 1-11-10 a.m. Did those experiences average five pounds per day?

Cymbalta, the last prescribed Alzheimer's disease medication, was discontinued. We no longer take medications prescribed for Alzheimer's disease. You will recall during the period of time when Jo was in Mercy Hospital in August 2008, Razadyne and Namenda were then discontinued.

January 11, 2010
Communication to CCDI Director:

Would Jo's treating physician order another chest x-ray to determine if water continues to appear?

To what extent does the thickener in Jo's water and juices and perhaps thickener in her puree or soft diet have on her digestive process, her urination, her water retention, bowel formation and its excretion?

What portion of the 2,000 cc of liquid daily is actually thickener?

What effect would or does Colace have on her digestive process, her urination, water retention, and bowel formation and excretion?

The combination effect of thickener and Colace?

It seems now that Jo usually has a large bowel movement every three or so days, if not by then a suppository is inserted. When she had a bowel movement before Colace, her stool was very large, at times it appeared two to three times the size of a hot dog weiner. It was amazing to me that she could excrete that sized stool. Subsequently, after Colace was prescribed, the stool has been very large, but it now appears as if someone ladled a large blob of peanut butter into the toilet bowl. It is presumed that continuous from 8-09-08 to date, a chewing and swallowing difficulty persists, therefore the continuing need for a soft diet.

After the treating physician receives a report from the CCDI care facility staff persons, after reading the above, what will be his prescribed orders for procedure?

Signed Claude Freeman, 1-11-10

July 6, 2010
Communication to the director of the CCDI care facility:

Jo is on a soft diet and thickened juices and liquids. Without Colace would those soft foods and thickened liquids harden during the digestive process?

163

Colace is a stool softener, which is prescribed to keep stools soft and easy, natural passage, and is not a stimulate laxative. Useful to constipation due to hard stools.

Colace is given to Jo every evening, mixed with applesauce, followed by thickened cranberry juice. Currently, her natural bowel movement is not too regular. Too frequently the softened stool is not passed naturally. Around the second or third day one or two laxative-type liquids are given, then if no bowel movement, a suppository is inserted, which normally results in a huge, peanut-butter-type substance being passed. The second and third days are tough on Jo, who noticeably endeavors to have a natural passage daily. Quite frequently, for a long period of time, a suppository has been used to empty the bowel of those huge wads of bowel that Colace has softened.

Soft food, plus a daily dose of Colace, a food softener. Is that good or bad? Should Colace be given every day? Should the prescribed dosage be lessened? Nature is endeavoring, but the softened consistency of the bowel must make it more difficult to have a natural passage. Please inquire of Jo's treating physician.

Recently, I have called to the attention of nurses and CMAs labored breathing of Jo. I would be sure there are notes to confirm. Each have checked her lungs, etc., which they report seem normal. Frequently, during our trips, spins, and visits in the evenings and during the giving of Colace, I notice the change in her breathing. Would the lungs now be retaining water, making it difficult at times to breathe normally? If not, what are the causes?

You mentioned recently, plans to walk Jo, and suggested I could assist by pushing the wheelchair behind the movement in event of legs wilting. Tell me the days and time of day. You may send a copy of this communication to Jo's treating physician if you elect.

Claude Freeman 7-6-10

Added note: Weight 1:25 p.m. 7-6-10, 171 pounds.
7-6-10, about 1:40 p.m.
Jo's treating physician ordered x-ray.

(I know Colace is referred to as a stool softener, rather than a food softener.)

Later in the day on July 6, about 1:40 p.m., Jo sitting on the stool, began an extra-large bowel movement, which process ended near 2:30 p.m. The individual bowel segments were huge, the bowel mass was incredible. A number of staff viewed the bowel in the stool, and were astounded.

July 9, 2010

I went to see Jo and was informed the treating physician gave instructions to continue Colace, ordered blood be drawn for two processes, ordered X-ray of chest and two x-rays of abdomen to determine if bowel is retained currently after large bowel movement on July 6 and bowel movement on July 8. The radiologist's findings reported on 7-9-10, among other things, "there appears to be marked distension of the stomach with air, large amount of stool seen in rectum. Obstructive pattern is not suggested at this time."

I have made notes of things related to me, which I endeavored to accurately retain, as follows:

Afternoon of July 8, bowel movement was on bed pads when Jo was checked.

July 10, I stopped by after 1:00 p.m., or so, and was informed Jo had a large bowel movement.

During my visit on the evening of July 10, Jo had no bowel movement success. She tried on the afternoon and evening of July 11, no success. In the morning of July 12, Jo was given prune juice, no bowel movement. On July 13, no bowel movement, even though Jo sat on the stool in the evening for 30 or so minutes. July 14, 5:00 a.m. or so, suppository was inserted. No bowel movement recorded at 10:00 a.m. or so.

July 14, 2010

Colace, suppositories, and bowel movement.

July 14, 2010

Memo to CCDI Director:

I have thought about the bowel cycle, about which we are all concerned. To get an accurate picture of the cycle, I am giving to the director of the CCDI facility a 2010 monthly monitor in which I request the director place by date, commencing 1-1-10, the first day that month a suppository was inserted in Jo and from and after that date record each date Jo had a bowel movement before the next suppository was inserted. Then record the next date a suppository was inserted, and from or after that record each and every date Jo had a bowel movement before the next suppository was inserted. I request that process be recorded up to the date the recordings are current, which I am certain, would be of great assistance to the treating physician and other medical persons he consults.

Signed Claude H. Freeman, July 14, 2010.

Requested a copy be sent to treating physician of Jo.

It is noted that between 7:30 p.m.-8:00 p.m. on July 14 she had a fairly large stool.

August 10, 2010

On Tuesday. August 10, a physician in the office of the treating physician of Jo left a message on my phone, in substance, that she and Jo's treating physician wanted to know how things were coming along. I elected to write the following, which I will fax first thing in the morning, Wednesday, August 11, 2010.

I know Jo continues at times to breathe somewhat labored. It appears her inhale is normal, but then her upper chest moves, which is not normal. It is more noticeable when she is being given Colace in

166

applesauce, after which she is given thickened juice. It is also noted, at times, when she is sitting on the stool in the bathroom and again, at times, when she is in bed, just before falling asleep. In bed, and before falling asleep, there is a little whistle-type noise as she breathes, which goes away when her bed is lowered and the head of the bed is at 45 degrees.

For some time I have noticed that Jo's right hand is colder than her left hand. The last few nights, for some reason, I felt her right forearm to determine if it was also colder than her left, and it was. We usually take a little spin in the wheelchair in the evening around the halls and, weather permitting, go outside to sit on the patio and talk and hold hands. Recently it has been very hot and humid, same experience, cold right hand.

Prune juice, bowel movement:

M-W-F prune juice at breakfast seemed to work quite well. Last Friday, August 6, Jo was given prune juice at breakfast; she then had a bowel movement in the afternoon. No bowel movement on Saturday, then on Sunday morning at breakfast (so called two-day-no-BM protocol) Jo was given prune juice. No bowel movement. Then on Monday morning August 9, Jo was given prune juice. Jo sat on the stool Monday night at bedtime for a long period of time, during which time she had a large stool movement. No bowel movement today, Tuesday, August 10, tomorrow morning, Wednesday, the 11th, Jo will get prune juice.

Soft diet feeding, portions are to be controlled.

Different persons spoon feed Jo at mealtimes. Does the pace at which spoonful portions are fed effect or affect the digestion process and bowel movements? During mealtime or at the end of the feeding process Jo is given the thickened juice and thickened water. Does excess liquid, juice, and water, during a meal or at the end of a meal before leaving the table have an effect or affect on the digestion process and bowel movements? With each spoonful of food given Jo at mealtime feedings, should the person feeding Jo tell Jo what is being fed, then, as food is placed in her mouth tell Jo to be sure to chew the carrots or sweet potatoes and then swallow? Would that process create for Jo a more normal feeding process, the chewing and swallowing and perhaps activating digestive juices which would cause more normal food processing and digestive procedure? There are in place instructions to not overfeed or stuff Jo.

Water retention now seems to concentrate from her armpits to her upper legs. Power hose M-W-F seem to be working from her knees down. Lotion and nightly massage of feet and ankles effective. Marvelous disposition, very cheerful, quite comprehensive and responsive.

Signed Claude Freeman, 8-11-10

Faxed to treating physician, copy to director of CCDI facility.

August 20, 2010

On or about this date, as I was preparing Jo for bed, I noticed redness in the middle of her chest which then extended left, under her arm and around to her back, splotches of redness which I called to the attention of the CMA on duty. A shower was given to Jo and after the shower, several of the red areas appeared to be glazed or have a blister-type appearance. This condition was then diagnosed as Shingles for which an anti-viral was prescribed (Acyclovir). Fortunately, there was no pain or discomfort and the condition was cleared rather quickly.

Just this past year I read in the Spring 2009 Alzheimer's *Research Review* (a publication for friends and donors of Alzheimer's Disease Research) an article entitled "Staying Healthy."

In the details of Jo's life, you can see that prior to the time she was invaded by Alzheimer's disease she had basically conformed to the principles being advocated in that article. The advice given in the *Research Review* follows:

The combination of social, mental and physical stimulation is the best medicine for a healthy life. It can also be a great way to avoid Alzheimer's disease. Even if you've been diagnosed with Alzheimer's, regular exercise and a nutritious diet can slow the disease's progress and help you cope with its effects.

Research indicates that staying mentally active can help slow memory loss and perhaps even lower the risk of developing Alzheimer's disease. Children and young adults build up brain "reserves" by reading and undertaking mental challenges, but older adults can build up their own reserves in similar fashion.

Among the mentally stimulating activities that can help form vital neural connections and buffer from cognitive decline:

- Learning to speak a new language
- Play a musical instrument
- Take up new hobbies
- Play board and card games
- Do crossword puzzles, brain teasers and word games
- Learning computer games
- Read books, magazines and newspapers
- Writing and corresponding through mail and e-mail

Other ways to provide mental stimulation include visiting museums, attending plays and even conversing and singing.

In addition to lowering the risk of high blood pressure, stroke and cardiovascular diseases, exercise can help prevent or delay the onset of Alzheimer's disease. Indeed, a new research suggests that exercise might actually break down deposits of toxic amyloid precursor proteins in the brain.

Consequently, scientists suggest a combination of aerobic exercise and strength and flexibility training, which will have the added benefits of improving overall physical and mental fitness, releasing stress and maintaining a healthy weight.

Scientists recommend a varied diet that includes vegetables, legumes (including beans, peas, and seeds), fruits, whole grain and fish. Avoid saturated fats and added sugars. Seek out foods with omega-3 fatty acids, including tuna and salmon, canola and olive oils, and nuts and seeds. And be on the lookout for foods high in antioxidants (vitamins C and E), including spinach, broccoli, cauliflower, berries, tomatoes, red grapes and carrots.

One knowing Jo Freeman as I did and had for 42 years would have never imagined that Jo Freeman would, in the latter part of 1999, begin to show signs of dementia, which signs did not cause real concern until a year or so later. Being realistic, and having read extensively about the onset of Alzheimer's disease, Jo and I have been coping with Alzheimer's disease for a total of eleven years, and probably longer. Together, over that period of time, Jo and I have learned Alzheimer's disease is very devastating for the person diseased, for the family, and for the primary caregiver.

Jo amazed me from time to time with remarks she profoundly voiced, after which statements or remarks I was highly elated.

After becoming a resident in a CCDI care facility, Jo continued to have acute hearing, and amazingly seemed to comprehend most things communicated in her presence when her attention was not distracted. She might not respond as expected, but there were times when her responses amazed those to whom her responses were directed, or who heard her responses.

Once when our daughter Susan was visiting and was present in the evening when it was time to get Jo ready for bed,

Susan sat in the bedroom area separated by a curtain as I was readying Jo for bed. As we were completing our process I said to Jo, "We did it," and Jo said in a very cheerful, animated voice, "And we did it together."

Jeanette, Jo's sister, was visiting, and Jo would listen to Jeanette and me as we endeavored to get Jo involved in a conversation, but Jo said very little. Jeanette decided it was time to leave, at which time I informed Jo I would see Jeanette out; as we walked away from where Jo was in a recliner, some 20 feet or so, we turned to wave goodbye. At that moment Jo said in a very clear, loud voice, "Tell everybody I said hello."

The activity director at the CCDI facility would inform me at times her surprise at Jo's unexpected comments. While she was reading the daily newspaper to residents, Jo was in a recliner at the time and appeared to be asleep. As the activity director read an article in which it was reported that some juveniles had been very destructive to property, Jo said, "Naughty, naughty." More recently the activity director informed me Jo had been very talkative and responsive at meal time and that she was so pleased Jo was that conversant. Later Jo really surprised her when Jo, very excitedly, said to her, "Let's you and I go play 18 holes of golf!"

One night at bedtime, as I was covering her up, I must have looked a little tired or sad. Jo said "I want you to smile!" I said I will, then she said, "I want to walk with you." I told her maybe we can walk tomorrow. Then she eagerly said, "I am counting on it."

On another night when I thought she was asleep, again in her excited or animated voice, she said, "Meet you for lunch tomorrow." One night a short while ago when it appeared Jo was asleep, she said in her animated manner, "See you early in the morning."

It has been tough at times, but man, how amazing, how impressive to observe that charming, animated bride of mine endeavor to, in her calm, quiet manner adjust to the progressive stages of Alzheimer's disease.

September 2, 2010

Correspondence to Jo's treating physician:

Re: Water Retention-Weight

Thank you for calling yesterday, 9-01-10, and communicating to me your observations after examining Jo, reviewing tests results, and after your discussions with the dietician at the CCDI facility.

I gleaned from your remarks, attention will now be given to fat, as water retention is not now a factor, at least not a serious factor. The only changes proposed was or is to increase Jo's protein intake, discontinue thickened juices, and I assume other thickened liquids, and substitute therefore juice and other liquids in which a prescribed amount of a powdered type of thickener will be added and stirred into the liquids given to Jo, which change in the thickening of the liquids fed to Jo daily would reduce Jo's daily caloric intake. Someone previously informed me the implemented thickening procedure would result in a reduction of 175 calories from Jo's current daily caloric count. In other words, Jo's current daily caloric count would now be 175 calories less than her previous daily caloric count.

If that process is continued and is adhered to daily, what is the expected weight loss per week or month? Did I hear correctly yesterday, one pound per month?

Weight has been a factor for some period of time!

For your information I will deliver to your office today, the following, concerning weight, diet, portions, and feeding, which subject matter I will endeavor to highlight with yellow marker.

Care Plan Conference Questionnaire Remarks, 10-11-09

11-05-09 Memo, copy of which was given to director CCDI care facility on 11-05-09

11-05-09 memo to director of CCDI care facility e: Jo's weight and meal portions

11-06-09 Diet and Weight, memo given to director of CCDI care facility, recreational director and dietician

11-10-09 Memo to dietician, director of CCDI facility and activity director

11-19-09 Memo to dietician and director of CCDI facility

11-19-09 Report from dietician re: Josephine Freeman

11-19-09 Attention all CNAs and Nurses from director of CCDI facility

[Note: the listed items sent to Jo's treating physician on September 2, 2010 are located in *Jo's Story* in date order.]

As you can see I inquired 7-14-09 "Why is Jo's weight so high, 155 lbs?" I now inquire, Why is Jo's weight so high, 171 lbs? Weight, diet, portions, and feeding? I do not want to hear sedentary! Everyone is aware that after breakfast she is put into bed for a couple of hours, then after lunch she is put into bed for a couple of hours; after dinner she does not usually get into bed until around 8:15-8:45 p.m. Those factors, including her inability to ambulate, and her history of bowel regularity, the texture of the bowel (frequently peanut butter appearance), the extremely large-content-sized bowel excreted should be taken into consideration when the necessary or required daily calories are fixed or determined. Were they? If so, should there be a review of conditions so that Jo's weight will not continue to increase beyond 171 lbs?

Claude Freeman 9-02-10

Copy will be delivered to CCDI Director

(Attachments to follow)

Care Plan Conference Questionnaire remarks dated 10-11-09 [found on page page 149 of *Jo's Story: Who Is Caring?*]

Jo's Story: Who Is Caring?

11-05-09 Memo, copy of which was given to CCDI Director:

Thursday, October 29, 2009, I had a brief inquiry of Activity Director as she was on the way to a meeting, and as we were talking the CCDI Director came out of the Director's office, and we posed a question to her. Her response was basically negative. I got home and thought I should inform the CCDI Director what had piqued my curiosity.

My inquiry re: Jo sipping through a straw came about after I had observed two or more days prior a cup sitting on Jo's lavatory in which was mouthwash-smelling substance, which piqued my curiosity! Could Jo now gargle and spit out the content? Could she sip juice after Colace-apple sauce was spoon given? Simple question?

Subsequently, I observed at a noon meal two different staff persons having Jo drink the juice from a glass tilted by that staff person. After the evening meal on the same day when I arrived I observed Jo's juice glass was empty; I inquired of the staff person if Jo drank all of her juice, and was informed yes, she drank it all. I inquired if she drank it from the glass, and she said yes, she did a good job. I was informed that is permissible, but sipping through a straw, no. Three months ago, 7-14-09, I noted in paper I wrote Jo's weight was 155 lbs, now 3 months later 10-09 she has gained 11 lbs to 166 lbs, some 40 lbs above her usual weight, 122-126 lbs.

Meals? Meal portions for each of the 3 meals per day—Saturday 10-31-09 saucer-sized (turned upside down) portion of tuna melt, cauliflower, assume cottage cheese—staff kept spooning in what was on plate—1/2 of the portions served would have been more than sufficient? Was the tuna, cauliflower, and cottage cheese thickened too? Jo always controlled her food intake, she naturally never stuffed, nor overate. Unfortunately, she is not aware presently the amount of food being placed into her mouth three times a day.

If all her three meals each day are of similar portions as served 10-31-09, plus thickened juice and water, are fed to Jo each of her meals daily, that is the cause of her weight increase.

WE HAVE TO LIMIT JO'S FOOD INTAKE! Otherwise she will not lose weight, weight gain will continue. Too much food may be a cause of large, difficult BM's, requiring Colace.

Met with the CCDI Director and Activity Director on Monday 11-2-09 re: weight and portions size, and feeding portions. This paper typed 11-5-09 from notes used in 11-02-09 meeting with CCDI Director and Activity Director.

Signed: Claude Freeman

11-05-09 Memo to CCDI Director re: Jo's weight and meal portions:

CCDI Director:
November 5, 2009
Re: Jo's weight and meal portions

Please provide to me this date, November 5, 2009, if you would please, Jo's highest weight recorded for each period of time listed below.

March 2007	135
March 2008	*144.5*
August 2008	*151*
March 2009	*147.5*
July 2009	*157*
August 2009	*159*
September 2009	*163*
October 2009	*164.5*
November 2009	*164*

As of this date November 5, 2009 have the three daily meal portions to be served and fed to Jo been reduced subsequent to November 2, 2009? *No, already receiving reduced portions.*

Since Jo is not ambulatory, and is basically sedentary, have all staff persons been informed Jo is not required or compelled to eat entirely all of the portions of food place before her? *Yes – discussed with nurses and CNAs*

Thank you for your consideration.
Signed by Claude H. Freeman 8:30 AM 11-05-09

11-06-09 DIET AND WEIGHT memo given to CCDI Director, Activity Director, and Dietician [found on ppage 155 of *Jo's Story: Who Is Caring?*]

11-10-09 Memo to Dietician, CCDI Director, and Activity Director [found on page 157 of *Jo's Story: Who Is Caring?*]

11-19-09 Memo to Dietician and CCDI Director [found on page 158 of *Jo's Story: Who Is Caring?*]

11-19-09 Report from Dietician re: Josephine Freeman [found on page 179 of *Jo's Story: Who Is Caring?*]

11-19-09 Attention ALL CNAs and Nurses from CCDI Director [found on page 160 of *Jo's Story: Who Is Caring?*]

September 27, 2010

A Meeting was scheduled for 1:00 p.m. with Jo's treating physician, Director of CCDI, and Dietician.

I, Claude Freeman, had prepared prior to that meeting a writing, which I read to those present at the conclusion of that meeting, as follows:

Each of you received a copy of my 9-2 letter directed to the treating physician, and received the attached referenced by date communications. Many questions were posed in those various communications. Many questions have not been answered as of this date. What are your answers and your proposed suggestions?

I see my wife sitting on the stool naked every Monday, Wednesday, and Friday night as I prepare her for her bath. I see her sitting on the stool naked every other night of the week as I prepare her for bed. Each of you would have concern as great as my concern if you personally viewed that body as I have for the past two years.

Jo has adjusted to the siege of Alzheimer's disease remarkably well.

She trusts me and you to keep her physically fit. She does not complain, even though she goes through great discomfort when her body does not function normally, such as food digestion and bowel discharge. She is aware of irregularities and remedies such as suppositories. Jo trusts people who give her care and when the caregiver's communication is soft and informative, she responds favorably.

Why did the water retention problem manifest? Once it was recognized and diagnosed, why hasn't it been treated, eliminated, cured? What are we doing now to eliminate and/or cure the condition? Are there too many people in the food preparation, portioning out the food, feeding Jo portions placed on her plate? Jo is given thickened water and juice a number of different times during the day. For breakfast, what thickened liquids are given Jo? Where and who mixed those thickened liquids? What thickener was used to thicken the liquids? Same questions regarding lunch, dinner, and in-between times when Jo is given additional liquids for hydration purposes.

Every night I am present when Jo is given Colace mixed in applesauce. We now have infrequent experiences when insufficient applesauce is mixed with Colace. Previously the thickened cranberry juice was predictable. Jo really liked that juice, it was very easy to hear her swallow that thickened juice. To lessen Jo's daily caloric count by 175 calories, that juice is no longer given. Now, cranberry juice is poured into a selected cup, and a powdered thickener is stirred into the juice, which viscosity is never the same. In fact, on most nights, it looks more like a gel and at times congealed in appearance like Jello. To Jo, I am certain she is aware of the difference, is this really cranberry juice? We (the CMA and I) hardly ever hear the swallow now. Previously, when we could hear the swallow, we knew Jo was ready for the next spoonful.

Last Saturday night, 9-25-10, there was no applesauce in the CCDI facility at the time the CMA was to start mixing the Colace with applesauce. A CNA went downstairs to get a supply from nursing. In the meantime, the CMA inquired of another CNA where the powdered protein was located. The CNA got the large, round container from the cabinet shelf and placed it on the counter. The applesauce arrived and was mixed with the Colace; the CMA then began to mix the thickener with the cranberry juice, then I witnessed the CMA put the powdered protein into a measuring cup, after which the CMA poured that protein into the thickened cranberry juice and began to mix it all together. As the CMA was mixing, I informed the CMA protein is never mixed as you are doing. I was informed instructions were to do as the CMA was doing. I noted white streaks in the mix which I knew was not what Jo was to be given after the Colace-applesauce mix was given. I suggested we not give the thickened juice-protein mix and requested we just give Jo more applesauce instead, which was done. Later, the CMA stopped me in the hallway and informed me the CMA owed me an apology—that after reading the instructions, the protein was to be given at mealtime, I believe.

Reduction of 175 calories in Jo's daily calorie count:

At what risks? Lessening that calorie count has not had any effect on weight (171.5 pounds). Water retention has noticeably increased in the thighs, hips, stomach, breasts, and now again, in the ankles.

Two or three Sundays past, I stopped around 1:15 p.m. to see Jo. When she finished her lunch I prepared her to go outside and as we were exiting, a very caring, alert CNA informed me I should have seen the plate set before Jo to be fed at lunch, which was twice as much as prescribed. The CNA then informed me the CNA took Jo's plate and removed by at least one-half the amount placed before Jo. That CNA informed me another CNA had been assigned to feed Jo that day, but when the knowledgeable CNA observed the size of the portions on Jo's plate, the CNA did as related above, for which aware-ness and action I thanked the CNA for being so observant.

Thursday night, 9-23-10, I arrived before Jo had eaten all on her plate. I walked over to her table to visually observe what was yet to be eaten and liquid to be consumed. I noted the food on the plate; the CNA feeding Jo informed me that a new person in the kitchen was serving food that night, and apparently did not know Jo was not to be served sweet potatoes. The CNA then informed me the CNA knew Jo was not to be served sweet potatoes and said I will not feed Jo sweet pota-toes.

November 19, 2009
The dietitian issued the following:

> *RE: Josephine Freeman*
> *The following measures were put into place:*
>
> *Breakfast meal would include*
> *½ cup hot cereal,*
> *One container yogurt,*
> *Nectar thickened liquids*
>
> *Lunch and supper meals would include:*
> *#20 level scoop of meat*
> *#20 level scoop of vegetables*
> *#20 level scoop of fruit*
> *Nectar thickened liquids*
>
> *No potatoes, rice or noodles are to be given. No casse-*
> *roles, bread or rolls or any other starch-type items are to be*
> *offered at any meals.*

Why did the kitchen person on Thursday night, 9-23-10 place on Jo's plate sweet potato?

Why did the CMA on 9-26-10 endeavor to give Jo powdered thickened cranberry juice plus a powered form of protein?

Knowledgeable alert people avoided mistakes referenced above. Obviously, all mistakes are not corrected before Jo is fed, or medicated.

Was there a request that Jo's treating physician be informed when Jo's weight exceeded 163 pounds, or a communication similar to that?

There was a pill given once or twice to get rid of water retained in Jo's system. Is there any way to reduce the water presently retained in Jo's system? Diet does not seem to be effective.

Forty pounds of additional weight is too much for Jo's legs, too much for her heart, too much for any body function!

As I said previously, Jo and I are dealing with the Alzheimer's disease quite successfully, but we are now faced with very serious body function conditions which we have little or no control over, for which conditions, the diagnosis of, treatment of, and care of, we rely heavily on each of you.

What will each of you do to alleviate or lessen the effect of the very serious body function conditions that currently exist?

Signed by Claude Freeman 9-27-10

Individual copies were given to the treating physician, the dietician, and the director of the CCDI care facility.

At the outset of that Monday, 9-27-10 meeting, the CCDI Director announced Jo's weight that day was 173 lbs!

October 1, 2010

On October 1, I went to see Jo at 1:45 p.m. I gave bra extensions to CCDI director in order that she could extend the length of Jo's bras. I noted Jo was in a wheelchair sitting in bad posture position; then waited for two CNAs to put Jo in bed for a nap. I noticed Hoyer lift being used.

10-1-10 Directed to Jo's treating physician by CCDI Staff:

1. Resident with increasingly labored breathing. Resident becomes Short of Breath with slightest exertion (eating, transfers, bathing) Blood Pressure this morning 139/84, Pulse 70, total this evening Blood Pressure 146/92, Pulse 54. Weights have been : 9/20: 173; 9/28: 173; 10/1: 171.5
2. We have an order to notify with each weight if resident weight over 165 pounds. Please advise

Order: No changes in orders (received from doctor 10-6-10)

10/01/10 Directed to Jo's treating physician by CCDI Staff:

Edema (swelling) to BLE (Bilateral Lower Extremities) 3 to 4 + (this means 3 to 4 times the normal), BUE (Bilateral Upper Extremities) 2 - 3 +. Trunk Edema (swelling) significant. Resident's skin (Bilateral upper and Lower Extremities, Trunk and Chest) is taut. Also noted that resident's urinary frequency total amount has decreased.

Order: Continue to follow (received from doctor 10-6-10)

10/04/10 Directed to Jo's treating physician by CCDI Staff:

1. Resident has a skin tear on Left forearm; circle size about 1/2 inch in diameter. Area cleaned, dried and edges approximated, steristrip (long strips of tape) applied, no swelling, warmth or pain indicated. Edges red no further current trauma to skin. We will continue to monitor.

2. Resident has increase in labored breathing during sleep. HOB (Head of Bed) elevated at 45 degrees at all times with feet elevated as well. Edema (swelling) +2-+3 BUE (Bilateral Upper Extremities). It was also reported that resident has had increased in drooling during meals and when given meals. Pox (Pulse Oximeter, measures oxygen in the blood) 92, RA (Room Air), T (Temperature) 97.6 degrees, P (Pulse) 60, R (Respirations) 13, BP (Blood Pressure) 152/86. Lung sounds are diminished BLL (Bilateral Lower Lobes).

(There are no orders on this report, just signed 10-6-10 acknowledging receipt thereof.)

October 2, 2010

I went to see Jo; she was sitting in chair slouched, dozing, tired. I inquired of the CNAs and CMA re: Hoyer use, the straps when not in use and placement of straps after Jo had been placed on the stool for bowel movement. They could not use the portable stool when Hoyer was in use as Jo's feet did not then touch the floor, or for some similar reason, so three

181

people would endeavor to lift Jo from the wheelchair via Hoyer, then lower her to the regular toilet seat in her bathroom, then detach the harness from the Hoyer, and spread the harness away from Jo's body parts so it would not interfere with her bowel movement efforts. There was a need for the CNAs to call the CCDI director for instructional clarification. I went home for dinner and returned around 6:15 p.m. Jo was not too energetic; Jo sat on stool about 30-35 minutes, just a tinkle and a bowel movement smear. The 3-11 p.m. staff was very responsive that night. I left about 9:15 p.m.

October 3, 2010

I went to early church; saw Jo about 9:00 a.m. sitting in wheelchair, Hoyer harness underneath her. I inquired re: toileting and learned she had wet the bed. The bed was wet when she was removed from bed to be dressed. She was not on toilet yet, had been given an early suppository. Around 9:25 a.m. or so CNAs put Jo on toilet seat. I sat with Jo for some period of time after which I pulled the cord for CNAs; lots of loud gas noise, some bowel movement, no tinkle. One CNA caused Jo to bend forward a bit, after which there was more gas expelled, some bowel movement. Jo was then placed in bed.

October 7, 2010

Jo was very tired, listless; two large bowel movements and one small bowel movement; took her Colace and applesauce; slow, not too responsive, only took one or two spoons of juice, no more. I sensed possible UTI.

October 8, 2010

I saw Jo about 1 p.m. and was informed by staff Jo took very little food or juice at breakfast; little or no food or liquids at lunch. I had a stronger sense of UTI so I requested a urine specimen, which was delivered to the lab at Mercy. Jo was taken to Mercy around 4:00 p.m. where ER staff gave extensive care and attention to Jo. After many tests, checks, and examinations, Jo was admitted and taken to a room at Mercy at approximately 11:00 p.m. where she was a patient from October 8 until she was transferred back to the CCDI on Tuesday, October 19, 2010.

October 9, 2010

I arrived early Saturday morning, the 9th, at Mercy, later a breakfast tray was brought to the room. An aide endeavored to get Jo to drink some juice and to eat to no avail. I noted a portable or movable elongated metal stand on which there were a number of plastic bags in which were liquids, nutrients, anti-biotics, protein, etc. Jo was very affectionate, but had a quizzical look as she tried to assess the environment. I noted a small cup of applesauce on the food tray and by spoon slowly fed most of the applesauce to Jo, telling her to chew and swallow.

About midmorning a partner of Jo's treating physician came to the room, which pleased me greatly. I had met him in August of 2008 when Jo was then a patient at Mercy. He, as he had in 2008, showed great concern and in detail outlined for me the ER report, which treatment was being implemented and what additional tests were scheduled, including that a swallow expert would be scheduled to determine why, for several days prior to her admittance, Jo had, for some reason, not spontaneously opened her mouth to receive liquids or food, and when she would, she would not then chew or swallow what was in her mouth.

October 10, 2010

Sunday, early church, then to Mercy. Jo not good, very tired, sleeping, no food, no liquids, except via tubes. Lasix was being given via tube. (I will note here that Lasix was continued for some time during this stay, and I noted her weight on admittance, and on discharge her weight was approximately 14 lbs less, as I now recall.)

October 11, 2010

Monday, the 11th, Jo no normal intake. The doctor I referred to above was on a four-day hospital assignment. He came in this morning and we had a lengthy visit about present care and treatment and alternative care and treatment upon release and transfer. During this visit I was informed that his partner, Jo's regular treating physician, was out of town and would be out of the country for some time and for that reason had not been in to see Jo. (I had not been informed by Jo's treating physician that he and his wife had those plans to be away.)

I had, in the meantime, talked with Jo's OBGYN, to whom Jo told her 16th tee world-upside-down experience to, and he agreed to talk with me, after which he agreed to familiarize himself with Jo's records at Mercy. Later he agreed to assume Jo's care.

Partners of Jo's treating physicians who assumed her care from day-to-day kept talking to me about tubes being implanted in either Jo's nose or stomach before her transfer back to CCDI. Then it was Saturday and Sunday, days I knew the CCDI director would not be in that facility. I knew then Jo would be transferred to the CCDI facility on Tuesday, the 19th. Monday I had a discussion with CCDI director. After that discussion, and a discussion with the OBGYN friend I determined there would be no tubes inserted in Jo's nose nor her stomach. She would be fully hydrated, medicated, nutritionally sated at the time of her transfer. Total peritoneal nutrition discontinued at 11:00 a.m. Tuesday, October 19, at which time she was transferred to the CCDI facility.

October 20, 2010

Lasix and antibiotics were prescribed and implemented on the 20th. Once or twice a CNA got Jo to consume some juice, no food. The CMA 3-11:00 p.m. got Jo to consume some juice twice, no food. I left about 9:00 p.m.; Jo was asleep.

October 21, 2010

Swallow expert came. She got Jo to allow her to put some juice, then applesauce in her mouth, little swallow, but mouth had to be cleared of residue. At 4:30 p.m. Jo was given some malted milk, no other liquid or food. At 8:30 p.m. she was asleep.

October 22, 2010

OBGYN to see Jo at 8:30 a.m. I visited with nurse re: Jo at dining table, placement and replacement in bed to avoid sores, feeding, oxygen mask, schedule, etc.

October 23, 2010

I visited Jo early. Jo was very affectionate, very loving; needs hydration; chair not a good experience; oxygen mask fitting at nose not good, closed her nostrils. CMA changed to fit for oxygen intake and normal breathing; placement in bed, rotation in positions timed, noted pillows under knees would cut off or reduce circulation, which was brought to CNAs attention.

October 24-28, 2010

Jo slept a lot; not too receptive of juice, but would sip milkshake now and then; was very affectionate, lovely bright eyes, smile, laughter; breathing labored; swallow expert here three or four times no success, no suggestions re: feeding or swallowing. CMA at 6:15 on 24th got Jo to consume some milkshake, then at 7:30 p.m. Jo became very awake, affectionate; Jo quite amazing.

October 29, 2010

At 9:30 a.m. very tedious, breathing very labored; 6:30 p.m. until I left at 9:00 p.m. the same. Earlier that day a CNA inquired if we had children to which I responded yes. The CNA then informed me it looked as if Jo was waiting for someone to come, very strong will to live. I thought about the CNA's observation as I tried to sleep and after waking the next morning the 30th.

October 30, 2010

I arrived to see Jo at 8:45 a.m. Saturday the 30th and observed Jo breathing very laboriously, very tense. She had been placed in bed specifically to avoid skin sores; pillows were placed to cause her to rest in a certain position, which positioning was changed approximately every two hours or so. I held her hand and advised her I was there. She would open her eyes and look at me, then with strong will continue the laborious breathing. I talked to Jo most all morning just to make her aware I was there, and as I talked I kept thinking about what the CNA had said yesterday.

As I talked with Jo, holding her hand, I asked her to let me see her pretty eyes, "open your eyes and give me that pretty smile," which she did, after which she continued to laboriously breathe. I then spontaneously began to inform Jo that I was all right, that Hugh and Susan were good, that we were fine; there was no need for her to be concerned about us, we were fine, and I said to Jo not to worry, that I was certain God had a special place for her, and she should not worry if she was ready, just let go, Hugh, Susan, and I would be fine.

The nurse in the room with Jo and I informed me it was time to reposition Jo. I left the room during which time the nurse and CNA repositioned Jo, and when they informed me I could come back into the room Jo was totally relaxed in her different bed position and her breathing was absolutely normal. She was completely at ease. I could not fathom or believe the change. I was so pleased to observe Jo so sedate, so calm.

I went home for a while, and upon my return after dinner I was informed by a CNA that she and another staff person had wakened Jo and they had just finished giving Jo a sponge bath, changed her gown, and other hygienic care. As the CNA and I walked into Jo's room I found Jo positioned in a relaxed, quiet manner, breathing in her normal effortless manner, for which attention and effort I thanked the CNA.

I sat down next to Jo's bed. She was sleeping quietly, firmly holding my hand. I communicated to her, but I am not certain if she was aware. I sensed a change in her being and I walked down the hall to request the nurse come with me to Jo's room, which she did. On arrival, she used her stethoscope to check Jo. The nurse stayed with Jo and I until Jo quit breathing. Life in Jo no longer at about 7:02 p.m., October 30, 2010, the night of the 11th day subsequent to her transfer from Mercy back to the CCDI facility.

WHAT A PARTNER! WHAT A SPECIAL LADY!

Subsequently, we received a great number of cards and personal expressions of individual experiences with, and memories of Jo, just a few of which I now share with you.

Charles and Peggy Strief: The Strief family always regarded it a pleasure to have been backyard neighbors to the Freeman family. This fund is a great tribute to Jo as were your words at the memorial service. Our thoughts are with you and your family.

Cathy Macomber: Dear Claude, I heard from Susan about Jo's passing. I know how devoted you were to her and also provided the best care one could give to her. I do remember all those great meals she prepared at 10 Lincoln Place and of course her laugh. Please take care of yourself, and I will be thinking of you.

Betty Koch: The service for Jo this morning was just right. A testimonial to a grand spirit with a special awareness of Alzheimer's disease. Jo was a real spark in the traveling "Honor Society." I will remember her with a smile.

Elise Hansen and Elise (Squeak) Geraghty: Dear Claude and Family, I just wanted to send our deepest condolences to you. I have many good memories of Jo, since I have known her for most my life and will always treasure them. You are doing a good cause to help continue the research for education to help insure excellent care of Alzheimer's victims. I am enclosing a check from myself and Mother to make a small endeavor for research. Thinking of you, Best regards.

Betsy and Kent Bro: Dear Claude, Jo was very precious. I am so sorry for your loss. We spent so much time together on the golf course and traveling to tournaments. She always would giggle and keep me positive. I also enjoyed her intellect and kindness. There will always be a warm place in my heart for her. Love to you, Betsy and Kent.

Anne Cownie: Dear Claude, Jo was one of my very favorite people and my thoughts and memories of her are very special. I always enjoyed being with her—especially in our Bible Study group—and at the bridge table. I admired her intelligence and her wit. You did a fantastic job at the funeral. I truly felt she was right there with us—and your eulogy unfolded like a beautiful love story. I will remember it always. You, and your family, will remain in my thoughts and prayers in the days and weeks ahead.

Sara (Johnson) Kinley and Ray: Dear Claude, our thoughts and prayers are with you and all the other members of your family at this time. You were truly blessed to have found such a wonderful partner in this journey of life. Your remarks yesterday were so touching and meaningful to all of us who know Jo—she was smiling! God bless her and may you find strength and comfort in your faith and love of your many friends and family members. Fondest regards.

Jack and Lois Watson: Claude, I admired your friendly wife and am so glad to learn more about her and her achievements. Lois and I will walk in your shoes, but we have compassion for you and keenly feel the loss you are experiencing. You have established a very special memorial for Jo with the Jo Hoyt Freeman Education Fund. We are pleased to make a small contribution knowing that the purpose of the memorial will help those who are working with patients like Jo and Lois to do an even better job of caring for them. It's a perfect tribute to Jo! Bless you, Claude!

Linda Zeiger: Claude, dear friend, Your love for Jo and her love for you was a beautiful example of God's love. I will treasure my friendship—the giggles—laughs—lunches—shopping—closet work—make-up and hair-do times we shared. I look forward to our heavenly reunion. God is with you at this difficult time.

Shirley and Ray Michel: Dear Claude and Family, We are grieved to learn of Jo's death. Her life touched ours in quiet ways—her interest in sharing a moment, her response of interest and engagement during an exchange of mutual interest whether it be a work of art, a knitting pattern or a golf game—and always her radiant smile. I'm aware of using the word "interest"—for me it was her great gift and one sorely missed these last years. She is included in my thoughts and prayers. God bless us all.

Di Findlay, Executive Director Iowa CareGivers Association: Dear Claude, I am writing to convey my condolences in the loss of your lovely wife, Jo. I also want to commend you for establishing the Jo Hoyt Freeman Education Fund for providing educational opportunities for direct care givers. Your act of love honors Jo and her passion for education and teaching, and it also raises the public's awareness about who direct care workers are and their need for more education and skill enhancement in the area of dementia care.

I would be happy to visit with you about your plans and to offer a little assistance in establishing the program in a way that will have an impact in areas that I think we both agree are very important. Once again, Claude, my deepest sympathies.

Brain Donation for Research
March 2006

I directed communications to two separate doctors in Des Moines on or about March 6, 2006, wherein I disclosed, in substance, "my wife resides in an ALP/D facility, an Alzheimer's unit. She recently expressed concerns of death, and matters to be addressed before. The other night when we were walking after dinner she suggested, in substance, giving her head to research, stating they can't find a cure for Alzheimer's, maybe it would help their research. She then requested I determine how one might do as she suggested.

"I turn to you, my friend, for that purpose. I enclose thoughts and questions that come to mind, which I would like to discuss with you when your schedule permits. Sincerely Claude H. Freeman."

I learned quite a bit reading Alzheimer's Society Dementia care and research's January 2005 sheet entitled "Brain Tissue Donations," including research centers for brain tissue donations: Boston University, National Institute on Aging; The Gerontological Society of America Re: Brain Donation in Normal Aging; Mayo Clinic; Washington University, St. Louis, MO; Northwestern University; University of Iowa, among others.

Responses were, in substance, as follows: "Generally, we prefer to do autopsies on patients whom we have seen as part of our research projects or if the person had been a patient. You are correct, Mr. Freeman, in noting that your wife would have to be a participant in the HOPE study before she would be allowed to donate brain tissue to the program. HOPE study participants must come to our center in Boston for annual examinations that last approximately four hours. So, it sounds like your wife would be ineligible for the study. This University Alzheimer's Disease Research Center has a brain donor program only for longitudinal research participants enrolled in the center."

I read neuropathologists are engaged to examine the brain tissue for evidence of Alzheimer's disease and pathological changes of other neurological disorders. I inquired through a long-time friend in Iowa City, in substance, if he knew a neuro-pathologist in Iowa City that had done or does autopsy on persons after their death to determine evidence of Alzheimer's disease and pathological changes of other neurological disorders. As time passed, being a donor to research in progress seemed unlikely.

Jo told one of her friends assisting her in recording "Jo's story" that: "Everything has gone stale on them. So I would be glad to give my head if they could come up with a cure."

Q. You mean when you die someday?
A. Yes.
Q. So that people could study and try to figure it out?
A. Yes, see this is the way it goes, we get so far and then we . . .
Q. See what we do is we talk about the different topics and then we can put them all together in order after we talk about them.
A. Yes, I see.

I presumed Jo might mention to our children her endeavor to donate her head for research and also inquire how susceptible they might be since Jo had been diagnosed as having Alzheimer's disease, followed by an inquiry as to autopsy. Those questions were not raised at that time, but to be prepared, and to do as Jo requested, in substance, determine who might examine her head.

I learned about the third week in March, 2006, there was no longer any Alzheimer's disease research done at the University of Iowa. I was also informed there were four neuropathologists at the University, two are clinical tract and two are research (muscle and cerebrovascular disease) but they do see surgical and autopsy cases as well. I was advised the neuropatholgists can do the brain removal and was given extensive information concerning the procedure process. On April 3, 2006, I directed a communication to the one neuropathologist who had answered my initial inquiries, to confirm I had determined "you should examine—study—the brain of my wife at her death; a brain-only autopsy. I will follow the prescribed instructions and cause to be implemented timely notices and changes."

Date and Time of Autopsy: 11/1/10 @ 9:30 Head only (brain)
  Final Autopsy Diagnoses
      I.   Diffuse Lewy Body Disease
           A) Fronto-temporal gyral atrophy
      II. Alzheimer's Disease, moderate
      III. Cerebrovascular Atherosclerotic Disease
           A) Focal acute ischemic changes
                1) Parietal lobule
                2) Deep nuclei
           B) Left middle cerebral artery territory infarct, remote
           C) Left head of the caudate infarct, remote
           D) Focal white matter ischemic damage, remote
           E) Moderate to severe arteriolosclerosis of the small
              and medium-sized cerebral and meningeal vessels.

IV. Diffuse contusions on the left lower shin (3/4 inch to 1 inch in greatest dimension)

Cause of Death: Complications of progressive dementia due to Diffuse Lewy body disease, Alzheimer's Disease, and cerebrovascular disease.

Other Significant Condtions: None

Manner of Death: Natural

Senile plaques are the histologic hallmark of Alzheimer's disease. These are seen in abundance in this case, confirming Ms. Freeman's diagnosis of Alzheimer's disease. However, numerous cortical Lewy bodies are also identified throughout the cortex. Lewy bodies can be seen in Parkinson's disease, however they are usually most prevalent in the midbrain in those cases. In cases where they are more widespread with no or little involvement of the midbrain, the disease is known as diffuse Lewy body disease. It is not uncommon to see accompanying Alzheimer's disease. Given the number and locations of the Lewy bodies seen in this case, it is the dominant form of dementia, set in a background of Alzheimer's disease and cerebrovascular disease.

Ms. Freeman's cause of death is best explained by complications due to progressive dementia. Diffuse Lewy body disease is the dominant pattern with accompanying Alzheimer's disease and cerebrovascular disease.

The manner of death is natural.

Subsequent to receiving and reading and absorbing the content of the autopsy report, I immediately retrieved my copy of the *Mayo Clinic Guide to Alzheimer's Disease* where I learned the following about Dementia with Lewy bodies (page 129).

The dementia type described in this chapter features distinctive structures call Lewy bodies—microscopic deposits of alpha-synuclein protein—found in deteriorating nerve cells. The existence of this protein buildup often cannot be confirmed until an autopsy is performed...

Dementia with Lewy bodies (DLB), with or without the presence of Alzheimer's disease, affects roughly 10 percent to 20 percent of people with dementia, making it one of the most common types of dementia... A few familial cases of DLB suggest that certain genes may be involved but so far, genes linked directly to the disorder have not been identified.

Alpha-synuclein protein normally is abundant in the brain, although its exact function is unknown. With abnormal function, deposits of alpha-synuclein build up within neurons to form Lewy bodies. The Lewy bodies become widespread (diffuse) throughout the brain as DLB progresses. In addition to the cognitive decline that characterizes most dementias, people with DLB usually have visual hallucinations and signs and symptoms similar to Parkinson's disease (parkinsonian symptoms), such as rigid muscles and slowed movement. These signs and symptoms fluctuate, especially in early stages of the disease.

Because the signs and symptoms of DLB are similar to those of other dementia types, particularly Alzheimer's disease, obtaining an accurate diagnosis is important. Some medications commonly used to treat psychiatric or parkinsonian symptoms may actually worsen the Lewy-body-related hallucinations and delusions.

Signs and symptoms:

...Cognitive impairment: The type of intellectual decline characteristic of dementia with Lewy bodies is marked by forgetfulness, attention deficit and difficulty following a single train of thought. The person appears disoriented and confused and often misidentifies people, including loved ones.

Psychiatric symptoms: People with DLB often have visual hallucinations involving vivid, colorful images of people and animals—although no sounds usually accompany the images. Some attempt to talk to or shoo away these perceived images, and they become upset if someone tries to convince them that what they see isn't real... Delusions, which are false beliefs, also are common with DLB. People may become paranoid and susceptible to conspiracy theories, believing, for example, that someone is stealing from them or that an impostor has replaced a spouse.

Motor symptoms. Some listed are: tendency to drool, balance problems, difficulty with refined motor skills, for example, handwriting or buttoning a shirt. The *Mayo Clinic Guide* goes on to say, "Although all these cognitive, psychiatric and motor symptoms are common with DLB, some people may never experience them during the illness. When they don't occur, it may be easy to mistake DLB for another type of dementia."

Sleep disorders. Particularly a condition known as rapid eye movement, also known as RBD, in which people appear to act out their dreams—also insomnia, sleep apnea, and restless legs syndrome.

Autonomic dysfunction. "In DLB, the autonomic nervous system—which controls involuntary muscle movements such as blood vessel, bladder and bowel contractions—is frequently impaired." This results in signs and symptoms such as: fainting, frequent falls, resulting from dizziness or fainting, impotence, urinary incontinence, constipation.

Diagnosis: "Doctors must diagnose dementia with Lewy bodies on the basis of the signs and symptoms described above. No biological test is available that positively identifies DLB—a definitive diagnosis is possible only at autopsy...DLB is often mistaken for Alzheimer's. Autopsies reveal that the brain tissue of most people with DLB also contains the characteristic features of Alzheimer's, such as amyloid plaques and neurofibrillary tangles, in addition to Lewy bodies. Doctors may refer to this combination as 'DLB coexisting with Alzheimer's disease.'"

"Scientists note that people with DLB who have few tangles tend to show primarily the symptoms of DLB, while those with many tangles exhibit symptoms closer to those of Alzheimer's. On the other hand, brain tissue of some people with Alzheimer's will contain Lewy bodies, even though no symptoms of DLB are apparent. This raises the question, still unanswered, of whether DLB and Alzheimer's are related in some way."

Treatment. "Because the underlying cause of dementia with Lewy bodies is still unknown, treatment is aimed at lessening the impact of symptoms on quality of life."

In this Mayo book, published in 2006, in the "Dementia with Lewy Bodies" section nondrug treatment, medications, anti-parkinsonian drugs, antidepressants, and memantine are discussed.

It's worth repeating how important it is to obtain an accurate diagnosis, ideally from a doctor experienced in treating dementia, such as neurologist or neuropsychiatrist. That's because some medications for treating general psychiatric and parkinsonian symptoms can actually make the DLB symptoms worse. The dosages and side effects of the various drugs must be continuously adjusted and balanced for optimal benefit.

Jo's Story: Who Is Caring?

Working for a Better Future

Di Findley, executive director, and John Hale, policy director, of the Iowa Caregivers' Association, have written a number
of articles that have appeared in the *Des Moines Register*. In
an article they wrote entitled "Care About Those Who Provide
Care," published June 14, 2007, they disclose "We, or someone
we are close to, will–due to age or disability–need the support of
a caregiver." It was published, "In Iowa, more than 60,000 people are professional caregivers, providing health care and long-
term care in nursing facilities, assisted-living centers, hospitals,
people's homes, group-care settings and other places.

"There's a looming concern about caregivers, though: The
supply of skilled professionals is dwindling at a time when the
demand for their services is greatly expanding." Findley and
Hale disclose that's happening for several reasons. "First, their
jobs are physically challenging and emotionally draining. Second, society doesn't respect them; too many of us look down at
too many of them. Third, they are poorly paid; many can earn
more in retail and fast-food outlets. And fourth, far too many
have inadequate health and retirement benefits, so they leave the
field for better benefits at another workplace down the road.

"The result of talented Iowans never entering or too quickly leaving the caregiving field? A decline in the quality of care.

"The lack of professional caregivers by health care and
long-term care has been called a crisis in the making. The aging

199

of baby boomers, it's been said, will produce a tsunami that wrecks havoc on the health-care and long-term-care systems. To a great extent, this reality is a wake-up call for Iowa."

EDUCATING THOSE WISHING TO SPECIALIZE IN THIS FIELD (ALZHEIMER'S DISEASE)

What criteria is one required to meet before that individual can be employed by an Iowa certified ALP/D or an Iowa certified CCDI care facility to provide and to give direct care to Alzheimer's diseased persons residing therein?

Are direct caregivers, that are not a certified RN, LPN, CMA, CNA or Activity Director, legally permitted to be employed in an Iowa certified ALP/D or a certified CCDI care facility to provide and to give direct care to Alzheimer's diseased persons residing there in?

No one should be employed in an Iowa-certified ALP/D or a certified CCDI facility as a direct care worker who has not successfully passed the required, prescribed, approved classroom education and hands-on training of how to provide care and support to those with Alzheimer's disease and their families.

It is obvious to many who have placed an Alzheimer's diseased family member in a care facility that the Director of Activity, RN, LPN, CMA, and CNA have had little or no classroom education and little or no hands-on training in their direct care of Alzheimer's diseased persons.

In "The Hub," Iowa CareGivers Association Newsletter: Special

Edition June 2008: Dementia Care in an article by Di Findley, Director, Iowa CareGivers Association, entitled "You Said You Need More Education on Dementia Care: Your Voices Have Been Heard," "As direct care workers (DCW)...You told us that you need and want more education and training on how to provide care and support to those with dementia and their families." Steps taken were listed by Findley, then in conclusion related: "You should feel good about sharing your voices. This is just one example of how you can have a positive impact on your career in caring and the quality of care you are able to provide to those you serve."

"Please watch the Hub and the ICA website for future information about this new education opportunity for direct care workers and other long term care workers."

In Senate File 2341 signed by Governor Culver 5-07-08, effective 7-01-08, Sec. 3, entitled IMPLEMENTATION: "The department of elder affairs shall implement on or before July 1, 2010, the initial provisions for expanding and improving training and education of those who regularly deal with persons with Alzheimer's disease and similar forms of irreversible dementia and for providing funding for public awareness efforts and educational efforts in accordance with section 231.62, as enacted by this Act."

What were and are the discussions on subsidizing educational opportunities?

How are the educational opportunities to be subsidized?

What educational opportunities would be subsidized?

Will the educational opportunities to be subsidized be defined better than "those wishing to specialize in this field"?

Subsidized education. When would paid-for education be most effective? (1) for those wishing to specialize in this field, or, (2) for certified Director of Activity, RN, LPN, CMA, and CNA who are direct care workers in a care facility where Alzheimer's diseased persons are residents, but which certified direct care workers have not been previously taught in a classroom setting nor have those listed had hands-on training on how to effectively provide care and support to the Alzheimer's diseased resident to whom they are currently attempting to give direct care to?

What criteria will determine the selection of persons to receive funds for the prescribed, approved, certified curriculum, and or courses of study?

What persons will be selected to receive funds for prescribed, approved, certified curriculum, and/or courses of study at designated approved, Iowa certified, learning institutions?

Who will determine what or which persons would be subsidized?

What curriculum or courses of study will the selected person(s) be required to pursue?

At what learning institutions will selected person(s) be permitted to pursue their education in prescribed, approved, certified courses of study?

Who will teach the prescribed, approved, certified academic

courses of study at the chosen Iowa certified learning institutions?

What curriculum, procedures, techniques, practices, communications, activities, environmental effects, et al., will be taught in the hands-on training process in the Iowa certified ALP/D and CCDI care facilities?

At what Iowa certified ALP/D and CCDI care facilities will the selected person(s) receive hands-on training of prescribed, approved, certified hands-on direct care of Alzheimer's diseased residents in Iowa certified ALP/D and CCDI care facilities?

Who will teach and instruct in the prescribed, approved, certified hands-on training courses of study at the Iowa certified ALP/D and CCDI care facilities?

Subsidized persons receiving and who successfully complete the required classroom course of study and hands-on training would then receive what certification?

For an Iowa certified ALP/D care facility what is the staff-to-resident ration requirement, if any?

For an Iowa certified CCDI care facility what is the staff-to-resident ratio requirement, if any?

What rule, law, or agency requirement specifies that ratio?

Between the hours of 8:00 a.m. and 8:00 p.m. the staff-to-resident ratio in an ALP/D care facility should be no less than a 1-to-5 ratio, excluding the activity director.

In a CCDI care facility that ratio should be no less than 1 to 4, excluding the activity director.

Direct care workers in ALP/D and CCDI care facilities shall not be required to launder resident's bedding or personal clothing, nor shall the direct care workers be required to plan, prepare, or cook meals for residents, or wash and dry implements used in preparing, cooking, serving, and feeding residents.

Usually direct care workers in ALP/D and CCDI care facilities work eight (8) hour shifts. Is the required staff-to-resident ratio the same of each eight (8) hour shift? If not, what is the required staff-to-resident ratio for each eight (8) hour shift?

What certified direct care workers, such as RN, LPN, CMA, CNA or others, are required to be on duty and present during each eight (8) hour shift?

The Iowa Department of Elder Affairs is, at the mandate of the Iowa Legislature, to develop new rules to enhance and expand dementia education requirements.

More Education and Better Training

The need for more education and better training is imperative. I learned this from personal experiences Jo and I had, from writing my "Alzheimer's Paper" and writing "Questions for Physicians." I also realized this after becoming familiar with the 2007 Alzheimer's Disease Task Force Final Report, and having many communications with Ann Riesenberg and Carol Sipfle, of the Alzheimer's Association, Greater Iowa Chapter, reading about the Dementia Education Preceptor Project and its well-received impact, learning of the enactment of Senate File 2341 and its intended purposes, reading very extensively and repeatedly, the content of "The Hub" Special Edition June 2008: Dementia Care, Iowa CareGivers Association Newsletter. I gained a better understanding from these experiences combined with other observations as well as excerpts from a transcribed discussion between my wife, Jo Freeman, and our friend Linda where Jo said: "Well they have tried but by the time they get settled so that they could start to take an exam, it is over. It is so late, they can't. Everything has gone stale on them. So I would be glad to give my head if they could come up with a cure."

Jo knew the importance of education when she was a student, then as an English, Latin, and French teacher her students subtlety came to know the importance of their individual education.

DCWs perceiving their need, and then publicly requesting

205

more education and training on how to provide care and support to those with dementia and their families confirmed DCWs should have that opportunity.

An awareness of all the above and knowing of the need for more education and better training caused me to sign and file on the 30th day of January 2009 ARTICLES OF INCORPORATION OF JO HOYT FREEMAN EDUCATION FUND, which was first publicly made known in Jo's obituary, published in the *Des Moines Register*, Thursday, November 4, 2010 as follows: "It was reported in the Iowa CareGivers Association Newsletter, 'The Hub,' June 2008 Special Edition: Dementia Care, in substance, direct care workers, 'You told us that you need and want more education and training on how to provide care and support to those with dementia and their families.'"

My interest in currently employed DCWs who perceive their need for, and who want more education and training has not waned subsequent to January 30, 2009, as you will see in the following communications.

July 14, 2009, Hale caused to be published in the *Des Moines Register* an article entitled "Health Care Won't Improve Without Enough Workers." Hale suggests, among other things, "Consolidate and update existing data on where work-force shortages lie. Capture data where it is incomplete, as is the case for millions of direct-care workers throughout America."

"Focus on common-sense solutions. Expand capacity (more space and more faculty) in higher-education institutions to train more medical professionals. Expand scholarships and loan-repayment programs for those who agree to practice in shortage occupations and locations... Expand mentoring programs and create career ladders that motivate newly hired direct-care workers to stay in their profession."

Carol Sipfle
Executive Director
Alzheimer's Association, Greater Iowa Chapter
1730 28th Street
West Des Moines, Iowa 50266

RE: 2009 Dementia Education Force

Dear Carol:

I extend congratulations to you, and to the Alzheimer's Association, Greater Iowa Chapter on being designated to serve as the lead agency in a collaborative effort with subcontractors, State Public Policy Group, Alzheimer's Association, Big Sioux Chapter, Alzheimer's Association, East Central Chapter, Alzheimer's Association, Midlands Chapter, and Iowa CareGivers Association to improve the availability and quality of dementia education for individuals in Iowa who care for people with Alzheimer's disease and related dementias.

I note that a Dementia Task Force consisting of stakeholders concerned about dementia education will be created to assist with revising administrative rules, develop a standard curriculum model, certify curriculum and trainers, create new curriculum when none exist for target audiences, and disseminate programs throughout Iowa. The Dementia Education Task Force will work closely with the Direct Care

Workers Advisory Council to coordinate activities, achieve common goals, and make use of limited resources.

I have prepared "Chronology for: 2009 Dementia Education Task Force," a copy of which CHRONOLOGY discloses the grave, pressing, imperative, need for a better academic, educational curricula, and live, hands-on training for future direct care workers who will become direct care workers in facilities where Alzheimer's diseased persons are residents. The CHRONOLOGY discloses more vividly the cry, and the urgency of the need for more education voiced by members of the Iowa CareGivers Association. ("The Hub"—Special Edition, June 2008)

I fax to you today, and to those noted at the conclusion of this letter, a copy of "Chronology for: 2009 Dementia Education Task Force," which CHRONOLOGY will be a good reference for you and members of the TASK FORCE as you commence your collaborative endeavors. I will provide additional copies you request.

Claude Freeman 9-03-09

FAX: Di Findley
     Heidee Barrett McConnell
     Ann Riesenberg

CHRONOLOGY FOR: 2009 DEMENTIA EDUCATION TASK FORCE

May 7, 2008, Governor Culver signed Senate File 2341, effective July 1, 2008.

Sec. 2. <u>NEW SECTION.</u> 231.62 ALZHEIMER'S DIS-
EASE SERVICES AND TRAINING.

3. The department shall adopt rules in consultation with the
direct care worker task force established pursuant to 2005 Iowa
Acts, Chapter 88, and in coordination with the recommendations
made by the task force, to implement all of the following training and education provisions:

a. Standards for initial hours of training for direct care staff,
which shall require at least eight hours of classroom instruction and at least eight hours of supervised interactive experiences.
b. Standards for continuing and in-service education for direct
care staff, which shall require at least eight hours annually.
c. Standards which provide for assessing the competency of
those who have received training.
d. A standard curriculum model for the training and education …
e. A certification process which shall be implemented for the
trainers and educators who use the standard curriculum model.

Sec. 3. IMPLEMENTATION. The department of elder affairs shall implement on or before July 1, 2010, the initial provisions for expanding and improving training and education of
those who regularly deal with persons with Alzheimer's disease
and similar forms of irreversible dementia and for providing
funding for public awareness efforts and educational efforts in
accordance with section 231.62, as enacted by this Act.

Direct care workers, caregivers, in care facilities where
Alzheimer's diseased persons are residents are begging for more
education on dementia care.

In the Iowa CareGiver's Association Newsletter, entitled
"The Hub," a Special Edition June 2008: Dementia Care, Di
Findley, Director, Iowa CareGiver's Association, caused an

article to be printed therein entitled "You Said You Need More Education on Dementia Care: Your Voices Have Been Heard." This special edition of "The Hub" is the result of a partnership between the Iowa Department of Elder Affairs (IDEA), Alzheimer's Association—Greater Iowa Chapter, and the Iowa CareGiver's Association. "You told us that you need and want more education and training on how to provide care and support to those with dementia and their families."

In that same issue of "The Hub" Special Edition June 2008, there is an article writted by Diane Frerichs, Certified Nursing Assistant (CNA), RNA, and Member of the ICA DCW Leadership Council, Co-Chair of the Iowa Direct Care Advisory Council, which article was entitled "Dementia Education Important for all Caregivers" wherein Frerichs writes, "You are waking up for the day. You are in a strange room and there is a stranger standing over you. How scary is that! There are 5.2 million Americans dealing with Alzheimer's disease each day, of this number 65,000 are Iowans. Every 71 seconds there is a new case. For many diagnosed with Alzheimer's this is just an example of what they face each minute of each day. Many are in Memory Care Units throughout the state and rely on Direct Care Workers (DCWs) to help them with their Activities of Daily Living (ADL's). These DCWs are required to attend 6 hours of Continuing Education each year to continue to work in these units. But there are also many of these residents with Dementia and Alzheimer's disease who are on the floor with the general population. Their caregivers don't have the added training to care for their special needs. The 2008 Direct Care Worker Task Force on DCW Education has recognized this need and will be recommending that there be added training for all new DCWs on Dementia and Alzheimer's—the disease and care of."

Findley reports in "The Hub," Special Edition June 2008

The following steps have been taken:

- You (DCWs) said you need more education and training in dementia care

- Iowa Legislature approved funding for the Iowa Department of Elder Affairs (IDEA) to test a dementia education preceptor program which was done in partnership with the Alzheimer's Association-Greater Iowa Chapter, and the Iowa Caregiver's Association

- Governor Culver appointed an Alzheimer's Task Force

- Alzheimer's Task Force met and made recommendations (report can be found on the IDEA's website: www.iowa.gov/elderaffairs/ or at ICA's website: www.iowacaregivers.org)

  - A direct-care worker testified at a Task Force meeting about the need for dementia education

  - Task Force recommended a special dementia care certification for DCWs and other long term care workers

- Iowa Legislature passed a bill that will fund the development of a special dementia certification to be administered through the Iowa Department of Elder Affairs

You should feel good about sharing your voices. This is just one example of how you can have a positive impact on your career in caring and quality of care you are able to provide to those you serve.

In the Dementia Education Preceptor Project (DEPP) final report filed July 2008 the following can be found on pages 12 and 13 thereof.

Continuation and expansion of the Dementia Education Preceptor Project brings with it several challenges:

Changing dementia education rules in Iowa—in 2008 the Iowa Legislature mandated that the Iowa Department of Elder Affairs develop new rules to enhance and expand dementia education requirements in Iowa. Continuation of this program should be put on hold until those new rules are finalized, as regulatory changes may impact this curriculum, the credentials of the instructors, program evaluation and other aspects of the project.

The Alzheimer's Association proposes convening a task force to explore these issues and develop a plan for expansion of the project. The task force would consist of representatives of Alzheimer's Association staff from all chapters in Iowa, the Iowa CareGivers Association, selected community college faculty and others. The group would work in tandem with the DEA (or its designee) as new dementia education rules are developed in Iowa.

The four education and hands-on training programs referenced in the July 2008 Dementia Education Preceptor Project Report were completed at the end of March 2008. Participants, preceptors, are now sharing their knowledge with co-workers in their respective places of work, such as nursing homes, assisted living facilities, and adult daycare centers.

As noted previously, in a book published by Alzheimer's Disease and Related Disorders Association in 1997 entitled *Key Elements of Dementia Care* (hereinafter referred to as KEOD 1997) it is pointed out that Alzheimer's/dementia care is unique and ever-changing.

Persons with dementia and their families have unique

needs; programs, environments and care approaches must reflect this uniqueness. As the field of Alzheimer's/dementia care continues to evolve so must our efforts to provide the best quality of care. Providers are encouraged to explore their commitment and grow to become "dementia-capable." Dementia-capable means skilled in working with people with dementia and their caregivers, knowledgeable about kinds of services that may help them, and aware of which agencies and individuals provide such services. This means being able to serve people with dementia, even when service is being provided to other people as well. Dementia-specific, on the other hand, means that services are provided specifically for people with dementia. On page 48 of KEOD 1997 under STAFFING ISSUES it is noted that not everyone is personally suited to work with persons who have dementia. The ability to operate effectively in a context in which roles are flexible and the focus is person-oriented instead of task-oriented is not universal. The ability to enjoy working under such circumstances should be identified among the requirements for employment in this field.

RECRUITMENT AND HIRING is a topic in KEOD 1997 at pages 52-53. Recruiting caregiving staff who reflect the qualities needed to provide dementia-capable care is definitely a learned skill. Working with dementia residents requires specific attributes and skills that go beyond a generic care program. Job descriptions and individual performance goals should include the values articulated in the program philosophy and mission statement.

(continuing)

Select caregiving staff for the special care program based on their experiences and commitment to the unique demands of caring for someone with dementia. Being successful in another area of the setting does not mean the individual is appropriate for the dementia care program. Find out if staff members want to work with residents with dementia.

Before transferring staff to a dementia program, be sure the staff feels the transfer is a reward for their hard work as opposed to punishment.

213

November 2008 IOWA DIRECT CARE ADVISORY COUNCIL made its "Report to the Iowa Department of Public Health Regarding Implementation of a System for Certification of Direct Care Workers."

On page 5 of that report it is noted, as required by House File 2539, this report includes recommendations to the Iowa Department of Public Health that build upon the recommendations provided by the Direct Care Worker Task Force established in 2005. "… As our residents and workforce age and retire, and consumers increasingly seek services in their homes, we must build a direct care workforce that is prepared to meet the needs of the future… Advisory Council Members embraced their role, and spent many long and intensive hours discussing elements of this new and innovative approach for credentialing direct care workers. Despite the numerous challenges faced by the Advisory Council, members found common ground in the need to develop a system for the future…"

At page 7 of that Report it is noted, "The Advisory Council was established in House File 2539 passed during the 2008 legislative session. The Advisory Council is charged with advising the Iowa Department of Public Health (IDPH) regarding regulation and certification of direct care workers. The work of the Advisory Council builds on recommendations from the Iowa Direct Care Worker Task Force that provides a framework for statewide standards for training and education for the direct care workforce."

At page 8, "The Recommendations of the Advisory Council build on recommendations from the Iowa Direct Care Worker Task Force that outline the following components of a new education and training system for direct care workers.

- Governance – This system will be governed by direct care workers themselves through the establishment of a professional board, much like other health professions. The board will have authority to certify workers and provide public protection.

- Standards for Education and Training – The Board will establish statewide standards for training and education of direct care workers, providing new professional opportunities for direct care workers by creating three levels of certified direct care workers. Certified direct care workers will also have opportunities to develop advanced or specialty skills through professional development and continuing education in areas of interest or associated with setting of practice or population served.

- Coordinated Instruction and Increased Capacity – As part of the development of standards for education and training, an accompanying training course for direct care worker instructors will be developed. The recommended structure will capitalize on the need expressed by employers to provide on-site training, but instructors will be certified so all training and education is recognized by the state."

At page 21 it is noted, "the standard curriculum is the foundation of this system, and therefore will need broad input to ensure that the training and education that will be provided meets the core needs of individuals that receive care and support from direct care workers. While stakeholders have been involved in development of competencies, disability interests continue to be underrepresented. These groups will be targeted to provide input that will ensure a curriculum that balances philosophy and practice across settings."

"Instructor training will be another element that requires input in Phase 1 to ensure that the network of instructors is appropriately trained to provide the broad education and training to direct care workers. The instructor network proposed for this system includes instructor trainers, primary instructors, and supplemental instructors. Some instructors will likely specialize and provide training as an employee of an agency or facility, but all instructors should have a level of preparation and knowledge that represents the diversity of settings and populations served by direct care workers."

At page 28, The Advisory Council expects to meet approximately monthly through June 20, 2009.

"Key activities for the Advisory Council in 2009 include:

- Continuing development and refinement of direct care worker core competencies, leading to the development of curriculum.

- Updating the Direct Care Worker Task Force Implementation Plan with grandfathering recommendations, communication and outreach recommendations, and time and resource estimates associated with technology, personnel, and partners for implementation. Recommendations provided in this report may have a significant impact on the overall plan for implementation.

- Supporting passage of legislation to establish the Board of Direct Care Workers within the Iowa Department of Public Health Bureau of Professional Licensure.

- Beginning outreach to stakeholders regarding the work of the Direct Care Worker Task Force and Advisory Council."

It is reported in the above-referenced Advisory Council Report at page 9 there are estimates of the number of direct care workers in Iowa which suggest up to 100,000 Iowans currently work in the direct care field. Direct Care Worker Advisory Council recommends "that, as with other professions, the existing workforce is allowed to transition as simply and seamlessly as possible into the new direct care worker education and training system.

"The Direct Care Worker Advisory Council recommends a regional phased-in approach to grandfathering the existing workforce... The Direct Care Worker Advisory Council recommends an established reporting and certification period of four years for grandfathering. During the four-year period, direct care workers who are working or who have worked in the direct care field during the previous five years will be eligible to report current education and experience and receive certification at a level that best matches their skills and job functions."

How many of those 100,000 currently working in the direct care field actually work in a certified ALP/D or a CCDI care facility, or work in a non-certified care facility where Alzheimer's disease persons are residents?

What percentage of those 100,000 direct care workers would resign or quit their job if they were assigned to give care to Alzheimer's diseased persons or persons with a related dementia?

The DEA issued a Request for Proposal in 2008: In the fall of 2008, the DEA informed the University of Iowa to proceed with its approved proposal; months later the State of Iowa instructed the University of Iowa to stop, and proceed no further.

If you are an RN currently employed in an ALP/D or a CCDI-type care facility where Alzheimer's diseased persons are residents, and you perceive neither you nor the direct care staff in that facility are adequately, properly trained in effective everyday communication with the residents nor properly trained in the physical, everyday needed hands-on care of the residents, where, how, and from what approved source can you, the RN, and the direct care staff become better educated, and more adept in effective communication and hands-on care of the residents in the care facility where you are currently employed? When and where can that RN and direct care staff, today, become better educated and receive greatly needed, live, hands-on training to which Alzheimer's diseased residents will be more receptive of or to?

Hands-on training would be most effective in a live, person-to-person, ALP/D-CCDI type residential environment. What persons, in Iowa, are qualified to give that person-to-person, live, hands-on training in every care facility in Iowa where Alzheimer's diseased persons are residents? When, where, and how can such gravely needed live, hands-on training, be implemented most expediently in ALP/D-CCDI residential-environment-type care facilities in the State of Iowa?

Currently, from an academic standpoint, who and where are the most capable, knowledgeable, competent individuals in Iowa concerning effective, everyday communication skills, with, and concerning effective, receptive hands-on care of Alzheimer's diseased persons who are residents in ALP/D-CCDI type care facilities?

Who or what schools, organizations or agencies provide currently, today, the requested advanced education and live, hands-on training?

CURRENT NEEDS MUST BE MET!

In "The Hub," Special Edition referenced above, Heidee Barrett-McConnell, Education and Outreach Specialist, Iowa CareGiver's Association, provided information for an article therein entitled "Education Small Steps Lead to Wonderful Destinations," wherein she relates:

Through DEPP, Dementia Education Preceptor Project, ICA had the opportunity to work with the Alzheimer's Association and share knowledge to approximately forty preceptors, who in turn serve as a resource person to their organization. The first ever curriculum that included a clinical component to the classroom education was a welcome prospect, one that was exciting and at the same time had the potential for many challenges. My experience in the clinical setting was remarkable. The student preceptors applied the morning classroom sessions to the afternoon clinical setting. Guidelines were developed to observe and to think about the individual person they were caring for and ways to think out of the box and become creative in care, to develop and provide additional person directed care, and to better understand the world of dementia.

This experience hopefully will open more doors and opportunities to learn and grow, to reach out and care for people with this disease and to provide the best quality of life we can give. Small steps lead to wonderful destinations.

Carol Sipfle, Director, Alzheimer's Association—Iowa Chapter, describes in the above-referenced "The Hub" publication the process through which the DEPP program was formulated, discloses sites where its educational and hands-on training programs were held, and expresses therein, due to the early success of the program and community college interest in making it an ongoing program, efforts are underway to repeat the program and expand it throughout Iowa.

In Sipfle's report the following appeared:

"This intensive combination of classroom instruction and hands-on experience is a unique approach to dementia care," said Ann Riesenberg, Program Director of the Alzheimer's Association, Greater Iowa Chapter. "We believe that allowing students to immediately apply the principles and concepts taught in the classroom to the actual care of persons with dementia will improve the quality of that care. It is also important to have role models and resources in dementia care settings to address the challenges associated with caring for those affected by Alzheimer's and related dementias."

The DEPP Program is a proven success.

The Alzheimer's Association, Greater Iowa Chapter, the Alzheimer's Association, Big Sioux Chapter, the Alzheimer's Association, East Central Iowa Chapter, the Alzheimer's Association, Midlands Chapter, and the Iowa CareGiver's Association could blanket Iowa with coordinated Demonstration Projects for Quality Dementia Education of Direct Care Workers. Trained personnel from each of the referenced Associations, utilizing the already prepared, tailored, effective DEPP primer or hornbook.

Direct worker attendees who become certified preceptors would then return to their Alzheimer's/dementia residential care facilities, and there better educate and train by example their colleagues in better communication skills, and more effective and more receptive communication skills, and better, more responsive hands-on skills.

This learned process would spread like wildfire among, and between the reported 100,000 direct care workers in Iowa.

The DEPP trained and certified preceptors are better educated and trained direct care workers; those trained and certified preceptors have a newly developed self-esteem; the care workers the preceptors train will also have a newly developed self-esteem, which care workers will then proudly and more effectively work each day to make life better in their Alzheimer's/dementia place of employment for themselves, and most importantly, for the residents therein.

CURRENT NEEDS MUST BE MET! Those needs must

be met immediately. Currently needs can be met through frequently scheduled Dementia Education Preceptor Projects (DEPP).

Once it is determined CURRENT NEEDS MUST BE MET, and those needs can and will be met immediately throughout Iowa, then financing of an approved DEPP-type program will be addressed.

The Alzheimer's Association, Greater Iowa Chapter will serve as the lead agency in a collaborative effort with subcontractors, State Public Policy Group, Alzheimer's Association Big Sioux Chapter, Alzheimer's Association Midlands Chapter, and Iowa CareGiver's Association to improve the availability and quality of dementia education for individuals in Iowa who care for people with Alzheimer's disease and related dementias.

A Dementia Education Task Force consisting of stakeholders concerned about dementia education will be created to assist with revising administrative rules, develop a standard curriculum model, certify curriculum and trainers, create new curriculum when none exist for target audiences and disseminate programs throughout Iowa. The Dementia Education Task Force will work closely with the Direct Care Worker Advisory Council to coordinate activities, achieve common goals, and make efficient use of limited resources. Finally, the project includes education and an awareness campaign for unpaid (family) caregivers.

> The Iowa Dementia Education Project Goal: Improve the availability and quality of dementia education for individuals who care for people with Alzheimer's disease and other related dementia.
>
> Objects of the Iowa Dementia Education Project: Create a Dementia Education Task Force consisting of stakeholders

concerned about the quality of dementia education in Iowa with the following purposes:

- Advise and assist the Iowa Dept. on Aging (IDA) with revising administrative rules to comply with SF 2341.

- Collaborate with IDA to develop a standard curriculum model as required by SF 2341 and certify existing training programs that comply with the standard curriculum.

- Collaborate with the IDA to certify trainers and educators of the standard curriculum model.

- Create new curriculum for expanded audiences (i.e. long-term advocates, law enforcement personnel, state surveyors and monitors) as required by SF 2341.

- Disseminate certified dementia education curricula to appropriate audiences within the timeframe of the project.

Collaborate with the Iowa Direct Care Worker Advisory Committee to coordinate its efforts on dementia education for direct care workers with the efforts of the Dementia Education Task Force.

Provide educational programs for unpaid (i.e. family) caregivers and conduct a public awareness campaign about the warning signs of Alzheimer's disease, importance of early detection, and availability of resources on Alzheimer's disease and related dementias.

Experienced, knowledgeable persons in the organizations funded, and the experienced, capable persons, stakeholders selected to serve on the to-be-created Dementia Education Task Force will fill and meet timely requirements and mandates set forth in Senate File 2341 because those selected are aware of, and they know the acute, voiced needs of the direct care workers, which needs were expressed in the June 2008 Special Edition of "The Hub."

Senate File 2341 is basically concerned about future Alzheimer's Disease Services and Training, which is to be implemented on or before July 1, 2010.

What about current needs?

What about the RN currently employed in an ALP/D or a CCDI-type care facility where Alzheimer's diseased persons are residents, which RN and Staff perceive they are not adequately, properly trained in effective everyday communication with the residents, nor properly trained in the physical, everyday needed hands-on care of the residents; where, how, and from what approved source can that RN, and the direct care staff become better educated, and more adept at effective communication and hands-on care of the residents in the care facility where they are currently employed?

No one knows better than the people in the IDA, the Iowa Alzheimer's Association, Chapters, the Iowa CareGiver's Association, and the direct care workers, their current needs for better education. Persons from the referenced entities will be, I assume, members of the Dementia Education Task Force.

The Dementia Education Task Force must discuss at length the direct care workers 2008 published need and want more education and training on how to provide care and support to those with dementia and their families. The expressed need and want included, I would be sure, better education on Alzheimer's/ dementia related diseases, training in effective communication skills and receptive hands-on care.

The Dementia Education Task Force must, more convincingly, make Iowa citizens aware of the prevalence of Alzheimer's disease, and its predicted ascendancy. Once the general public in Iowa is made aware of the prevalence and predicted ascendancy of Alzheimer's disease, then Iowans can be informed of the direct care workers need and requests for more education and training on how to provide care and support to those with dementia and their families. Once Iowans are made aware of the prevalence and predicted ascendancy of Alzheimer's disease, and direct care workers recognized need and requests for a better education re: Alzheimer's/dementia related disease, better communication skills, and training in hands-on direct care of Alzheimer's/dementia diseased persons, those informed and then concerned citizens in every town, city, and county in Iowa, and people in their churches, organizations, and service clubs will raise necessary funds to pay the cost of better eduation and training direct care workers currently employed in their locales to give direct care to and for Alzheimer's/dementia related diseased spouses, family members, friends, and other persons.

The Dementia Education Task Force must give time and thought as to how, when, who can and who will schedule and present a DEPP-type program in their town, city, or county!

CURRENT NEEDS MUST BE MET!

Signed by Claude H. Freeman, 8-24-09

The Association entered into a contract with the IDA in July 2009 to implement the requirements of SF 2341. A project was developed with an overall goal to improve the availability and quality of dementia education for individuals who care for people with Alzheimer's disease and other related dementia. The Association began work on the project in August by creating a dementia education task force to develop training standards, create new curricula, and disseminate programs throughout the state. The task force represented a diverse group of stakeholders, including individuals from various healthcare and social service disciplines, settings at which care is provided, educational institutions, caregivers, and others. The task force held its first meeting in September to begin its work and formed sub-committees to address specific projects. Initial work also occurred on a statewide public awareness campaign and six regional education conferences for family caregiver conferences.

In October, Governor Culver signed an executive order requiring state agencies to reduce their budgets by 10%. Consequently, the funding for this project was reduced from $182,350 to $72,517. See Appendix A for a summary of work completed prior to October 31, 2009. The project was inactive from November 2009 to January 2010 as the Association and IDA awaited confirmation of funding and then scaled back the project to align with available funds. A revised contract was signed in early February 2010 and the project resumed shortly afterwards.

Revised Goal

Improve the availability and quality of dementia education for direct care workers who provide care for people with Alzheimer's disease and other related dementia.

September 15, 2010, the *Des Moines Register* published an article by John Hale entitled "Care Workers With Low Skills? Hardly." Wherein Hale discloses that too many Americans value the work done by direct care workers yet remain comfortable with them living in near-poverty status. They say such things as, "I could not do the work they do," "They are angels," and "There's a special place in heaven for people who do this work."

My response to those comments is this: Thanks, but giving them a special place in heaven doesn't keep a roof over their heads, put food on their tables, clothe their children, pay their medical bills, make the car repairs, etc. It's hard to do that on $9, $10 or $11 an hour and working all too often without adequate health insurance. That's why so many of them leave the work they are ideally suited for in order to do easier, higher-paying work with better benefits at a factory, office, or so many other workplaces.

Who is going to care for Mom or Dad or the child with a disability or someday you? If we don't begin to change the way we view and treat critically important people, the answer may be no one, or someone who is unqualified to do so.

In the Iowa CareGivers Association Newsletter: "The Hub" Special Edition June 2008: Dementia Care, the following was published:

The Need for More Education on Dementia and Alzheimer's Disease

In gathering information for the Alzheimer's Task Force work, the Iowa Department of Elder Affairs heard the need for both public and professional education repeated over and over again from families, consumers, caregivers, health professionals, and others.

Research findings reported by the Iowa Better Jobs Better Care Coalition and AARP Iowa support the need for more dementia specific education and training.

- Only half of the Certified Nursing Assistants (CNAs) who have worked in a Chronic Confusion and Dementing Illness (CCDI) unit report that they have taken the required 6-hour Alzheimer's/CCDI training course.

- Only about two-thirds of CCDI administrators/licensed nurses believe that the required 6-hour Alzheimer's training course prepares CNAs to provide high quality dementia care.

"The Hub" Special Edition June 2008: Dementia Care!

My how I wish this publication had come into my hands back in 2006 when Jo was a resident in the ALP/D facility! I have referred to this publication many times herein, but again another reference is helpful in communicating care to be given Alzheimer's diseased persons.

Ann Riesenberg, then Program Director Alzheimer's Association—Greater Iowa Chapter, wrote an article entitled "Difficult Symptoms...Problem Solving Strategies" wherein I extract and relate to you the following:

There are many symptoms that can occur with someone who has Alzheimer's...It can be very helpful for caregivers to try and determine why the person with dementia is behaving in a certain way. This may lead to identifying ways to prevent these difficult symptoms from occurring again.

Potential causes for difficult symptoms can usually be grouped into four categories:

- Physical or emotional problems like depression, constipation, pain, fatigue or the effects of certain medications
- Environmental issues such as excessive stimulation, clutter, poor sensory environment, or a space that is unfamiliar or too large
- Causes related to the task if there are too many steps, or if the task is not modified for increasing deficits or unfamiliar to the person with dementia
- Poor communication which can lead to not being able to make needs known or to understand what is expected of them

...Keep in mind... the person with Alzheimer's is trying to communicate...it is not happening because the person is stubborn, nasty or trying to irritate you!

Riesenberg also wrote in the same June 2008 Special Edition an article entitled "Dementia Care...No Matter What You Call It," wherein she related the following:

There are many names applied to models of care for persons with Alzheimer's and related dementias... What do these various approaches have in common?... Each person has a unique life history, values, attitudes and traditions. However, the person with Alzheimer's does have the same feelings and emotions as someone who does not have the disease. Affection, recognition, empathy, dignity and feelings of self-worth are basic needs for a person impacted by Alzheimer's.

...Direct care staff who are successful care providers for people with Alzheimer's are not task oriented but person oriented. They know the life story of the person for whom they are caring.

Also published in that Special Edition are:

Tips on being a Successful Dementia Care Provider:
- Empathize and recognize what the experience of Alzheimer's disease is like for those affected.
- Know the abilities of the persons that you care for and pay less attention to what they are unable to do for themselves.
- Understand the basics of Alzheimer's disease as a foundation for good caregiving skills.
- Know the life stories of the people for whom you care.
- When a problem arises, remind yourself that many behaviors result from attempts to communicate needs and cope with the world of Alzheimer's.

Basic Communication Techniques in Dementia:

- Approach the person slowly from the front; speak only when he or she can see you

- Remove all distractions—shut off television, music and radios

- Position yourself at eye-level with the person

- Keep your interactions one-to-one

- Use words sparingly; gestures, pictures, pointing to objects are helpful

- Give the person time to respond (at least 20 seconds before you repeat your message)

- Repeat yourself using the exact same words

- Always maintain a smiling face and a gentle tone of voice

Mike McCoy, a longtime friend of Jo and I, sent to me a *New York Times* reprint article dated December 31, 2010 by Pam Belluck entitled "Giving Alzheimer's Patients Their Way, Even Chocolate," in which article it was disclosed that the care facility, Beatitudes, referenced in the article, is in Phoenix.

Margaret Nance was, to put it mildly, a difficult case. Agitated, combative, often reluctant to eat, she would hit staff members and fellow residents at nursing homes, several of which kicked her out. But when Beatitudes nursing home agreed to an urgent plea to accept her, all that changed.

Disregarding typical nursing-home rules, Beatitudes allowed Ms. Nance, 96 and afflicted with Alzheimer's, to sleep, be bathed and dine whenever she wanted, even at 2 a.m. She could eat anything, too, no matter how unhealthy, including unlimited chocolate. And she was given a baby doll, a move that seemed so jarring that a supervisor initially objected until she saw how calm Ms. Nance became when she rocked, caressed and fed her "baby," often agreeing to eat herself after the doll "ate" several spoonfuls.

...Ms. Nance, in her wheelchair, happily held her baby doll, which she named Benjamin, and commented about raising her sons decades ago. Ms. Alonzo had at first considered the doll an "undignified" and demeaning security blanket. But Ms. Gallagher explained that "for a lot of people who are parents, what gives them joy is caring for children."

"I was able," Ms. Gallagher said, "to find Margaret's strength." Ms. Gallagher said she learned when approaching Ms. Nance to "look at her baby doll, and once I connect with the doll, I can look at her."

She squatted down, complimented Benjamin's shoes, and said, "You're the best mom I know."

Ms. Nance nodded earnestly.

"It's good to know," Ms. Nance said, "that somebody knows that you care."

Ms. Nance sensed she was then in an environment where someone cared about her, she was in an environment where the people there focused on individualized care.

Read the article you will find the epitome of *Jo's Story: Who Is Caring?*

When I first read the article, it kind of reminded me of the elating experiences Jo had with Linda, Deb, and others when writing *Jo's Story*, and reminded me of Jo's positive relation with the nurse, acting as activity director, prior to that person's departure 5-09-06. I also reflected on Brawley's book wherein Brawley pointed out there are seniors who are bored, helpless, and lonely in facilities all over the country, which means we urgently need to move beyond the medical model of care and embrace a more social model that focuses on the individual in a meaningful, life-affirming way.

I also reflected on a more recent experience, one which occurred at the CCDI facility late summer of 2010, which I allude to herein elsewhere: More recently the activity director informed me Jo had been very talkative and responsive at meal time and that she was so pleased Jo was that conversant. Later, presumably that day, Jo really surprised her when Jo, very excitedly, said to her "Lets you and I go play eighteen holes of golf!"

The following is a quote from the above-referenced Belluck article: "'In the old days,' Ms. Alonzo said, 'we would find out more about somebody from their obituary than we did when they were alive.'"

That quote would suggest staff in a facility where Alzheimer's/dementia diseased persons are residents learn all they can about each resident, get to know them, help them be who they were and really are; let each separate resident know you are interested in them individually, that you care about them, which in turn the resident will instinctively perceive, and confidently within themselves conclude or form a mental impression "this person is interested in me, knows things I have done or things that interest me; here is a person I can communicate with, this person cares about me." Soon the DCW realizes the resident's self-esteem, self-confidence, self-worth have improved, the resident is more relaxed, more his or her natural person or being. The DCW will then be so motivated and stimulated to continue to assist the Alzheimer's/dementia resident to be as receptive as Ms. Nance was. As the saying goes, the better staff knows the resident, the better staff can cause and allow the resident to be his or her natural being— prime example, Ms. Nance.

Memories Slip, but Golf Is Forever

Mike McCoy sent to Jo and I another article, which was published Wednesday, April 8, 2009, in The *Wall Street Journal,* entitled "Memories Slip, but Golf Is Forever," by Matthew Futterman, wherein, among other things is was reported:

> Anyone who has dealt with people suffering from mid-to late-stage Alzheimer's knows how difficult it can be to transport someone from fear and confusion to contentment and lucidity. But at Silverado [Senior Living home in Belmont, Calif.], caregivers have stumbled onto a technique that works nearly everytime—a golf outing. They run through a series of putting drills, knocking the ball around with the wonder of small children playing the game for the first time, which is how many of them experience it each week. For those who played the game when they were younger, swinging a club often sparks a startling transformation, however fleeting, that can make them seem like regular old folks again.
>
> Experts in Alzheimer's say these weekly golf outings illustrate an individualized method of an increasingly popular treatment known as behavioral therapy. Behavioral therapy has been around for more than a decade, but personalizing the treatment to a patient's interests is less common. Rather than providing the same series of experiences to every patient, caregivers have begun to search for activities patients enjoyed when they were younger, and to allow the patients to experience them again. "This is motor memory for these people, and usually you don't lose that," said Carl Cotman, a professor of neurology at the University of California at Irvine.
>
> ...Silverado and other assisted-living facilities often use activities like dancing or playing music to stimulate their residents. Like golf, such activities have proved helpful in both making people with dementia feel competent and generating periods of lucidity.
>
> The rule for memory among brain specialists is "first in, last out." The things we learn first—our names, for instance—are the memories we hold on to the longest. John Daly, director for the geriatric medicine fellowship training program at the University of California at San Diego, said explicit memories—what you had for breakfast or even the

current appearance of a spouse or a child—are stored in the cerebral cortex. Alzheimer's usually affects this part of the brain first. Skills like swinging a golf club or playing a musical instrument are part of what is referred to as implicit or procedural memory, which is centered in the cerebellum and other areas of the brain. These are often some of the last memories Alzheimer's patients lose.

Push Alzheimer's sufferers to remember or recognize things they no longer do, and they will often become agitated, as most people do when they are being forced to understand something that is confusing. But give them an activity that once brought about true pleasure, and the agitation can dissipate, their minds can clear, and memories related to that activity can return.

...for Joan Brown, an elegant, 82-year old Alzheimer's sufferer, the chance to hold a club and putt for a while is like a powerful mood-altering drug. Ms. Brown's son, Steven, moved her to Silverado last year because she kept wandering away from the assisted-living facilities where she had been staying. She needed a place where the staff would monitor her 24 hours a day. Last Wednesday morning, terror gripped Ms. Brown at the thought of heading out for an afternoon of golf. "I can't do that," she said, shaking her head and growing agitated. "I've never played golf before... No, I can't do that at all."

...But just after noon, as Ms. Brown and her son began tapping balls toward their targets on the putting green... she spoke of how she had learned to play as a child in Calgary, Canada. Her father, a Scot, was a committed golfer, she said. She recalled taking lessons from a local pro and talked about the weekly ladies rounds she played. "I could always hit the ball long," she said. Noticing a few small dogs on a leash nearby, she remarked that they weren't allowed on the golf course, and that the managers probably weren't too happy about them being there. When one of her 10-footers rolled into the hole, she looked up with bemused surprise and batted her blue eyes. "Oh," she said, "such perseverance."

Another wonderful example of caring!

Caregiving is a continuous learning experience.

How does a caregiver find the key to unlock stored memories of activity in the brain of an Alzheimer's/dementia diseased person, which activities once brought about in that person true pleasure?

Caring Skills

I was made aware in 2006 persons caring for Alzheimer's/dementia diseased persons need special skills to care properly for those diseased individuals.

You have previously read in *Jo's Story: Who Is Caring?* about budget cuts, reduction of funds, changes in administration, departmental changes subsequent to the June 2008 Special Edition: Dementia Care publication.

The JO HOYT FREEMAN EDUCATION FUND was established in honor of my wife, Jo Hoyt Freeman, an Alzheimer's/dementia diseased person who in her progressive diseased condition related in *Jo's Story: Who Is Caring?* "I have a story to tell...I want to be one of those good citizens who want to improve your and my lives by helping. One step at a time."

Articles of Incorporation of the JO HOYT FREEMAN EDUCATION FUND were filed in the Office of The Secretary Of State Of Iowa January 30, 2009.

Jo Hoyt Freeman died October 30, 2010.

Subsequent to Jo's death I have labored hard to write *Jo's Story*. All net proceeds from the publication of *Jo's Story: Who Is Caring?* will be used for the purposes for which the EDUCATION FUND was established.

For more information about the Jo Hoyt Freeman Education Fund, and how you may contribute to the Fund, please see the Jo Hoyt Freeman Education Fund section that follows.

The DCWs who perceive, and publicly make known their need and want for more education and training on how to provide care and support to those with dementia and their families cause me to believe those who make known their need for more education and better training tacitly imply their intent to continue to give care and support to those with Alzheimer's/dementia diseases and their families.

The curriculum must be designed to teach the skills DCWs personally perceive they need, and teach the skills advocated by Riesenberg in her articles referenced in "The Hub," and skills disclosed in the *New York Times* and the *Wall Street Journal* articles referenced herein.

COMMUNICATION SKILLS and HANDS-ON CARE TECHNIQUES ARE IMPERATIVE!

Jo Hoyt Freeman Education Fund

Contributions to the **Jo Hoyt Freeman Education Fund** are greatly appreciated. Your contribution should be directed to GREFE & SIDNEY, P.L.C. Attorneys at Law, 500 East Court Ave, Suite 200, P.O.Box 10434, Des Moines, Iowa 50306. AT-TENTION Thomas W. Carpenter or Robert C. Thomson. Make checks payable to the "Jo Hoyt Freeman Education Fund."

The **Jo Hoyt Freeman Education Fund** was established in honor of my wife, Jo Hoyt Freeman. ARTICLES OF INCOR-PORATION OF JO HOYT FREEMAN EDUCATION FUND were filed in the Office of the Secretary of State of Iowa January 30, 2009. My intended endeavor, January 30, 2009, and now the personal endeavor of the Directors of the Jo Hoyt Free-man Education Fund, is to work with the Iowa Alzheimer's Associations, Iowa CareGivers Association, and various edu-cational institutions to create an approved learning curriculum, to be taught in scholastic learning environments, and in Al-zheimer's/dementia care facilities where Direct Care Workers (DCWs) will receive advanced knowledge about Alzheimer's/ dementia diseases, and be taught better, more effective com-munication skills, and individualized care methods. Their Al-zheimer's/dementia diseased residents will then be more recep-tive of, and more favorably responsive to the newly acquired methods of communication and individualized care.

The Board of Directors of the **Jo Hoyt Freeman Education Fund** are as follows: Claude H. Freeman, President and Direc-tor; Roger F. Grefe, GREFE Capital Management of

RAYMOND JAMES & Associates, Inc.; David L. Brown, Lawyer, Hansen McClintock & Riley Law Firm; Mike McCoy, Insurance Executive, Arthur J. Gallagher Risk Management Services, Inc; and Tom Leahy, Lawyer, retired, formerly associated with Claude H. Freeman at Grefe & Sidney.

Acknowledgments

In June of 2010 I compiled a bound volume entitled "Alzheimer's Disease, Who Is Caring?" This volume included articles I had written, newspaper articles clipped from the *Des Moines Register*, correspondence I had written to persons, correspondence received in response, as well as specified pages from the June 2008 Special Edition on Dementia Care of "The Hub" (Iowa CareGivers Association Newsletter, "Dementia Education Preceptor Project (DEEP) Final Report Summary").

I met with and gave a bound copy of "Alzheimer's Disease, Who Is Caring?" to Robert A. Burnett, MEREDITH CORPORATION CHAIRMAN AND CEO RETIRED, on or about 6-24-10. Subsequently, Bob returned the manuscript, and related to me that I had done a workmanlike, thorough job, and then suggested I consider enlisting the help of a writer who has the knowledge and skill to deal with a project of this kind. Bob informed me he had contacted such a person.

Through Bob I came to know Sylvia Miller, former magazine editor at MEREDITH CORPORATION.

Sylvia looked at and read the bound chronology, then suggested, among other things this was not in a "book" format. I visited with Sylvia and she agreed, as time moved forward, to read and type volumes of material I presented to her, which became *Jo's Story*. The effort of Sylvia, her observations, suggestions, and comments I greatly appreciate.

In Section 3 of *Jo's Story: Who Is Caring?* you will read a paper I wrote, then signed January 12, 2007, a copy of which I mailed on March 26, 2007 to Jim Hayes, an Iowa City attorney whom I had known for a long period of time. In that letter I informed Jim that the paper had been widely circulated in areas of Iowa; I inquired of Jim, after he had read the paper, whether or not he would have in mind any person who would "make a difference," as I would like for some strategic person(s) in the Medical School to get a copy. He led me to Kitty Buckwalter.

Kitty has a PHD in nursing and was a professor of nursing at the UI College of Nursing, specializing in gerontology. I came to know Kitty, and learn through frequent communication of her interests and efforts. On August 1, 2011 I met Kitty in person at Jim's office in Iowa City, on which occasion I gave to Kitty a rough copy of *Jo's Story*. Kitty, though retired, and many in the Iowa Geriatric Education Center, the University College of Nursing, and I believe the Hartford Advisory Board will be greatly pleased to see that *Jo's Story: Who Is Caring?* has been published. Jim, especially Kitty, and all of her associates, who have worked constantly and diligently with Kitty in utilizing *Jo's Story*, and in efforts to get *Jo's Story* published, I greatly thank you.

Now that *Jo's Story: Who Is Caring?* has been published, almost verbatim as it was written in 2011, I hope and trust Kitty and her colleagues will use this publication now for purposes they perceived.

Robin Findley, secretary for Tom Carpenter and Bob Thomson, at my old LAW FIRM, Grefe & Sidney, P.L.C., has been of great assistance over the past few years typing, copying, mailing items, making suggestions, being a good sounding board, and most of all offering encouragement in my endeavor to cause *Jo's Story: Who Is Caring?* to be published. I also thank Tom and Bob for permitting Robin to do as she has over that time span, which I greatly appreciated.

I thank Scott Edelstein for directing me to Patti Frazee, a publishing consultant who read *Jo's Story, Who Is Caring?*, and after reading that manuscript met with me personally to discuss the contents thereof, and the manner or form in which *Jo's Story* is presented. Patti gave me the opportunity to relate to her why I chose a chronological presentation of the story. This chronological presentation of diagnosis and personal experiences is beneficial not only for spouses and loved ones it will be especially beneficial to their doctors treating their loved one, doctors selected to diagnose their loved one as the disease progresses, and will be especially beneficial to students in medical school who will in the future have patients who present with a benign memory loss. The chronological presentation will be an elementary text or a primer for the above referenced, as well as for students learning to be care givers of Alzheimer's/Dementia Diseased persons, and also beneficial to those direct care workers currently employed in ALP/D and CCDI facilities who want to be better educated and trained.

Patti, I greatly appreciate your interests, your inquiries, your thoughts, and ideas, but most of all, you listened. Patti you are a very professional person, a one in a million!

In July 2012 I met Bruce W. McKee, Patent Lawyer, Des Moines, Iowa, for lunch during which I requested counsel and advice in my effort to publish *Jo's Story: Who Is Caring?* Bruce agreed to provide that advice and counseling. Bruce informed me subsequently, there will be no charge for my assistance as this is an important charitable project. Bruce, I thank you for your effective counseling, personal effort, and for being so magnanimous.

Bibliography

"2010 Alzheimer's Disease Facts and Figures," Alzheimer's Association, http://www.alz.org/documents_custom/report_alzfactsfigures2010.pdf, Washington D.C.: 2010.

"Adequate Food and Fluid Consumption," Alzheimer's Association Greater Iowa Chapter News, 2006, pp. 9-10.

"An Exciting New Target for Alzheimer's Therapy," Alzheimer's Research Review, A Publication for friends and donors of Alzheimer's Disease Research, Summer 2009.

Barrett-McConnell, Heidee. "Education: Small Steps Lead to Wonderful Destinations," "The Hub," Iowa CareGivers Newsletter, Iowa Caregivers Association. Special Edition June 2008: Dementia Care.

Belluck, Pam. "Giving Alzheimer's Patients Their Way, Even Chocolate," The *New York Times*, December 31, 2010.

Brawley, Elizabeth C. *Design Innovations for Aging and Alzheimer's: Creating Caring Environments*. Hoboken, NJ: John Wiley & Sons, Inc., 2006.

"Campaign for Quality Residential Care," Alzheimer's Association Greater Iowa Chapter News, September 2006.

"Could a Spice Help Prevent Alzheimer's Disease?" Alzheimer's Research Review, A Publication for friends and donors of Alzheimer's Disease Research, Fall 2009.

"Dementia Education Preceptor Project," Contract #0820, Final Report, Alzheimer's Association, Greater Iowa Chapter, July 2008.

Findley, Di. "You Said You Need More Education on Dementia Care: Your Voices Have Been Heard," "The Hub," Iowa CareGivers Newsletter, Iowa Caregivers Association. Special Edition June 2008: Dementia Care.

Findley, Di and John Hale. "Care About Those Who Provide Care," The *Des Moines Register*. June 14, 2007.

Fischman, Josh. "Alzheimer's Today," *U.S. News and World Report*, December 11, 2006.

Frerichs, Diane. "Dementia Education Important for all Caregivers," "The Hub," Iowa CareGivers Newsletter, Iowa Caregivers Association. Special Edition June 2008: Dementia Care.

Futterman, Matthew. "Memories Slip, but Golf Is Forever," The *Wall Street Journal*, April 8, 2009.

Hale, John. "Care Workers With Low Skills? Hardly," The *Des Moines Register*. September 15, 2010.

Hale, John. "Health Care Won't Improve Without Enough Workers," The *Des Moines Register*. July 14, 2009.

Iowa Department on Aging, *Elder Affairs (321)*, Chapter 25, "Assisted Living Programs" (2004).

Iowa Department of Inspections and Appeals, *Inspection and Appeals (481)*, Chapter 58, "Nursing Facilities," (1999).

Iowa State Senate, *An Act Relating to Alzheimer's Disease and Similar Forms of Irreversible Dementia*. Iowa Senate File 2341, effective July 1, 2008.

Key Elements of Dementia Care. Alzheimer's Disease and Related Disorders Association, Inc., 1997.

McCalley, John. "Dementia Care: A Priority for the Culver Administration," "The Hub," Iowa CareGivers Newsletter, Iowa Caregivers Association. Special Edition June 2008: Dementia Care.

"New Report Reveals Impact of Alzheimer's Disease in Iowa," Alzheimer's Association Greater Iowa Chapter News, Spring 2010.

Petersen, Ronald, M.D., Ph.D., ed. *Mayo Clinic Guide to Alzheimer's Disease: The Essential Resource for Treatment, Coping and Caregiving.* Rochester, MN: Mayo Clinic, 2006.

"Pitting One Protein Against Another," Alzheimer's Disease Research flyer, rev: 1/10.

"Report to the Iowa Department of Public Health Regarding Implementation of a System for Certification of Direct Care Workers," Iowa Direct Care Advisory Council. November 2008.

Riesenberg, Ann. "Dementia Care...No Matter What You Call It," "The Hub," Iowa CareGivers Newsletter, Iowa Caregivers Association. Special Edition June 2008: Dementia Care.

Riesenberg, Ann. "Difficult Symptoms...Problem Solving Strategies," "The Hub," Iowa CareGivers Newsletter, Iowa Caregivers Association. Special Edition June 2008: Dementia Care.

Sipfle, Carol. "Dementia Education Preceptor Project (DEPP)," "The Hub," Iowa CareGivers Newsletter, Iowa Caregivers Association. Special Edition June 2008: Dementia Care.

"Staying Healthy," Alzheimer's Research Review, A Publication for friends and donors of Alzheimer's Disease Research, Spring 2009.

"The Need for More Education on Dementia and Alzheimer's Disease," "The Hub," Iowa CareGivers Newsletter, Iowa Caregivers Association. Special Edition June 2008: Dementia Care.

"Tips on Being a Successful Dementia Care Provider," "The Hub," Iowa CareGivers Newsletter, Iowa Caregivers Association. Special Edition June 2008: Dementia Care.

To Order Jo's Story,
go to Amazon.com, other online retailers,
or
order a copy from your local bookstore.